THE INTEGRATED PRACTITIONER

Food for Thought

BOOK 5 OF *THE INTEGRATED PRACTITIONER* SERIES

JUSTIN AMERY

Radcliffe Publishing
London • New York

Radcliffe Publishing Ltd
St Mark's House
Shepherdess Walk
London N1 7LH
United Kingdom

www.radcliffehealth.com

British Library Cataloguing in Publication Data

A catalogue record for this book is available from the British Library.

ISBN-13: 978 184619 776 5
Volume set ISBN-13: 978 184619 950 9

The paper used for the text pages of this book is FSC® certified. FSC (The Forest Stewardship Council®) is an international network to promote responsible management of the world's forests.

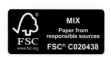

Typeset and designed by Darkriver Design, Auckland, New Zealand
Printed and bound by Hobbs the Printers, Totton, Hants, UK

Contents

Contents

These books are dedicated to my Dad, Tony Amery, who was a wonderful doctor and who is still my inspiration.

About the author

I am a full-time practising family practitioner and children's palliative care specialist doctor working in the UK. I have also spent some years working in Uganda and other sub-Saharan African countries.

I enjoy teaching, writing and mentoring. I am a medical student tutor at the University of Oxford, a trainer in general practice, and I have designed and set up children's palliative care courses for health professionals in the UK and Africa. I have worked with 'failing practices' to help them turn round; and also with health professionals who are struggling (as we all do from time to time).

I have always had an interest in philosophy and spirituality, and have studied this at postgraduate level. I have carried out some research into education and training of health professionals around the world and I continue to explore that interest.

I have previously written two books: *Children's Palliative Care in Africa* (Oxford: Oxford University Press, 2009) and the Association for Children's Palliative Care (ACT) *Handbook of Children's Palliative Care for GPs* (Bristol: ACT, 2011). I particularly enjoy reading and writing poetry.

At heart, though, I am a practitioner and a generalist. What is more, as you can probably see, I am rather a jack of all trades, and a master of none.

I have been motivated to write this book as I am hoping to explore practical ways of practising health that help us all, patients and practitioners alike, to become a little more healthy, and a little more whole.

Acknowledgements

These books have been brewing up over many years and so there have been very, very many influences upon them. There are far too many people to mention and thank without risking leaving someone out, so I shall just mention those who have been immediately involved.

Firstly, thank you to those very kind and patient people who helped review the drafts and gave such helpful feedback: Maria Ward, Penny Thompson, Meriel Lynch, Tom Nicholson-Lailey, Peter Burke, Penny Moore, Susan McCrae, Caitlin Chasser, Louise Rutter, Polly Steele, Rachel Samson, Laura Ingle and Maddy Podichetty.

I would also particularly like to mention Chris Smith, who not only gave very useful feedback on these books, but who also helped me to develop a lot of the ideas in them through his leadership of the Oxford Advanced Consultation Skills Course that I help him with, and over a few pints in the pub as well.

Thanks as well to Gillian Nineham of Radcliffe Publishing, who was brave (or daft) enough to put her faith in these rather unconventional offerings; suggest numerous areas for improvement and offer tremendous support and encouragement in their publication. Thanks also to Jamie Etherington and Camille Lowe for all their help in putting them together.

I would like to thank my colleagues at Bury Knowle Health Centre in Oxford, Helen House Hospice in Oxford, Hospice Africa in Kampala, Uganda, and Keech Hospice in Luton. They have all shown utmost patience and perseverance as I have led them on various merry dances, contortions and deviations in the name of 'good ideas', rarely reminding me of the 99% which failed, and always supportive of the 1% that, miraculously, did.

Of course I can't forget Karen Bateman (the doctor) and Karen Amery (the missus) who has been a continuous and never-ending source of sound advice, support and wisdom.

Finally, I would like to offer a huge thank you to Polly who, on a cliff top in Spain, gave me the courage to risk writing this stuff down and making it public.

Introduction to the series

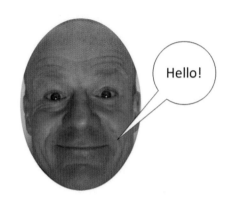

Hello!

Hello and welcome! This is me. You and I will be sharing a journey through this book, so you may wish to know what I look like. Because practice can't happen without practitioners, I will be popping up now and again, to test-drive some of the ideas that we will be discussing.

WHY ARE THESE WORKBOOKS NEEDED?

If you are, like me, a modern-day practitioner, you are probably still dedicated to the idea of good practice, but feeling rather buffeted by many and various winds of change that are sweeping through. You are also probably feeling (like me) that it would be good to have two minutes to sit back and reflect a little: to think about what's working and what's not; and maybe even to find a little balance.

If this is how you feel, you have come to the right place. So welcome!

In this series of workbooks we will be doing exactly that, taking a little time out, thinking about what we are doing, looking at things from different perspectives and using different lenses, and trying out some practical ways of making our practice more effective, more efficient, and (above all) more satisfying.

On the other hand . . .

If you are, like me, a modern-day practitioner, you will probably also be moving far too quickly to have any time for doing anything except what you need to be doing. In other words, you probably don't feel you have time for luxuries like sitting back and thinking. Frustrating though it may be, you probably have time to do only what you *have* to do, rather than what you *want* to do.

If this is how you feel, you are still in the right place, so welcome again!

In this series of workbooks, we will be working under the clock, recognising that there are boxes to tick and targets to hit. No doubt you don't just need to keep up to date, you need to prove you are keeping up to date too, for appraisal, or for review, or for revalidation. So, as we go along, we will be providing practical examples that will help you not just to reflect upon but actually to develop your practice.

What's more, we will even be providing appraisal certificates, so our appraisers, line managers and bosses will stay happy too!

But you're gonna have to serve somebody, yes indeed
You're gonna have to serve somebody,
Well, it may be the devil or it may be the Lord
But you're gonna have to serve somebody.

– Bob Dylan

WHY DID I WRITE THEM?

I have written these workbooks because there doesn't seem to be anything out there that scratches my itch. Our experience of real-life health practice is messy, complex and often chaotic. It doesn't seem to bear much resemblance to the practice we read about, or even the practice we try to teach our students and trainees.

Modern scientific and philosophical understandings of the universe are complex, messy and relational too. But our models of health and health practice often seem to be built on glib and simplistic models, or they fall into dualistic discussions (for example, about 'patient-centred' or 'practitioner-centred' care; or about 'traditional' or 'alternative' practice; or even about 'disease' and 'health'). Is the world really like that?

I have also written these books as I am worried about the levels of demoralisation and burnout among students, trainees and colleagues that I meet, right across the globe. Of course we can all get a bit tired, burnt out, and maybe even ill. If we are honest, we are often sceptical and occasionally a little cynical about what we do. But if we are even more honest than that, at heart we believe in what we do, because we think it is important.

It's not that we want to turn the clock back. We can feel a considerable (if quiet) sense of pride in how far health practice has developed. But perhaps we'd also like to think that, in the 21st century, there is a way for our practice to include and yet somehow to transcend what has gone before. It's not that we want to reject the practicalities, the science, the technology and the politics. On the contrary, I think most of us wish to accept and value them. But we also want to do what evolution always does: including, building upon and then transcending what has gone before. In so doing, maybe we can also rediscover the art of what we do, and perhaps even find a way of expressing ourselves with a little more poetry.

WHAT WILL BE IN THEM?

The answer to that is simple really. We are hoping to look at practice from different perspectives, and using different lenses, so each book takes a different view.

- Workbook 1 – *Surviving and Thriving in Health Practice*. We are the foundation of everything we do. Without us there would be no health practice. We are our own most useful tools. So, in the first book, we will look at how we can keep ourselves sharp, surviving and thriving in practice.

- Workbook 2 – *Co-creating in Health Practice*. As practitioners, whenever we come into contact with our patients, we create something very familiar but also very strange: a relationship. This relationship is neither me nor the patient, but some sort of third entity, which has an existence of its own, partly from me, and partly from the patient. This 'co-creation' is arguably our most powerful tool, but it is a tricky one to use. So we will focus on that in the second workbook, considering how we might practise in a way that co-creates healthier and happier existences, for both our patients and ourselves.

- Workbook 3 – *Turning Tyrants into Tools in Health Practice*. As practitioners we have a vast array of tools that we can use: time, computers, money, information, colleagues, equipment, targets, our workplaces and so on. If they get out of balance, however, each of these tools can become a tyrant, so that it has control of us, rather than the other way round. So in workbook 3 we will be looking at some of the most important tools (and tyrants), considering how we can stay in control of them (and not vice versa).

- Workbook 4 – *Integrating Everything*. Health practice is, ultimately, a single integrated thing. While workbooks 1–3 have been looking at the different 'bits' of this 'whole', workbook 4 is where the rubber hits the road, because it is here that we try to put it all together and come up with ways that we can integrate everything into a happier, healthier and more skilful whole within the real-life, complex and messy world of health practice.

- Workbook 5 – *Food for Thought*. We are practitioners, so we are practical, and interested in practice. So we will leave the theory until last. But most of us like a little bit of theoretical background to give context to, and to underpin our practice.[1] So workbook 5 tries to provide that. Everything that exists does so against a background. Indeed the word 'exist' means to 'stand out'. All of our experiences, beliefs and understandings of health practice derive from a living, organic and constantly moving context: whether scientific, philosophical, cultural, aesthetic, biological or spiritual. It is useful therefore to spend a little time understanding and reflecting on these building blocks of who we are. As practitioners, we don't always have time to do this, so we will leave this book until last. It will be a little luxury for those with a little more time, not essential, but hopefully a bit nourishing. Like a fireside cup of cocoa.

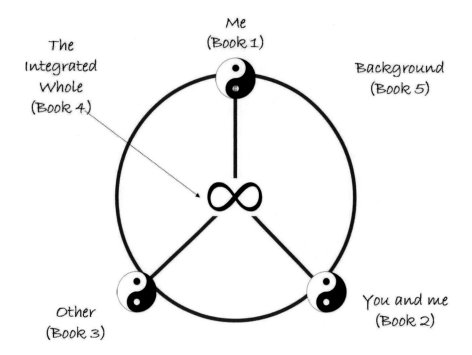

WHAT PERSPECTIVES AND APPROACHES WILL THEY USE?

In the 21st century we practise healthcare in a strange tension.

Science has taught us that we live in a highly relational, messy, multidimensional, complex, blurry and even chaotic universe. The humanities and philosophy have taught us that much of what we hold to be 'true' is relational and cultural and socially constructed. The arts teach us the value of creativity and expression in all walks of life. Spirituality teaches us about perspective, the value of awareness, and the fundamental interconnectedness of all things.

However, despite this relationality, creativity and complexity, we seem to be practising in a world that seems ever more bound and codified, with ever more targets and tick boxes, according to models that seem unrealistically geometric and two-dimensional, and with ever less room to breathe and to express ourselves.

So, in these workbooks, we will try to be practical and pragmatic. While we may not necessarily like the rules, regulations, guidelines, laws and targets that have nosed into our practice, we recognise that they have their uses. We know that health is a political football, and we are used to being kicked around a bit.

As practitioners in the 21st century we also value (and sometimes worry about) the advances that science and technology have brought. As practitioners, we are scientists, and we have a duty to do our best to ensure that what we do is as safe and effective as possible. We recognise that finding an evidence base for what we do is important not just for safety, but for development too.

So in these workbooks, we will start from the premise that we should, wherever possible, look for empirical evidence for what we are suggesting. On the other hand, we will remain vigilant to the blind spots of the empirical and technological approach, and look for alternatives to fill any gaps that we find.

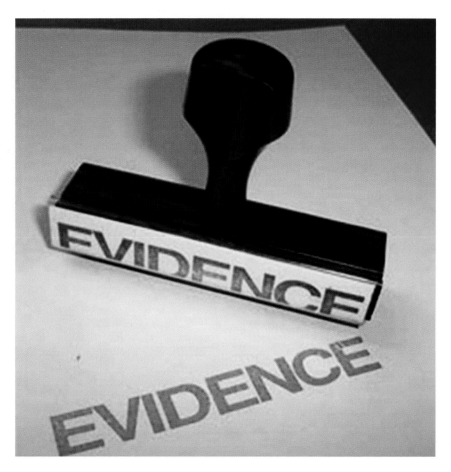

Wherever possible we will look for empirical evidence for what we are suggesting.

As modern practitioners we are scientists, and also technicians, but we are artists too. There is an art to being a practitioner, and in fact practice is an art. We might lose sight of it sometimes, but we are in the business (and busy-ness) of trying to create healthier and happier existences for our patients, and hopefully for ourselves too.

So in these workbooks we will be using plenty of imagery, art and illustration to engage the more creative sides of our brains, and to remind us that integrated practitioners need to be able to find balance between creative and practical.

These days, we don't tend to talk much about spirituality. Many of us would not think of ourselves as 'religious', and some of us might be horrified at the idea that modern-day practice should have anything to do with spirituality.

But most of us perhaps like to feel that there is some purpose or meaning behind what we do. We may hope that our practice connects with and somehow reflects the values and traditions of our families as well as of our broader societies and cultures. We deal with life and death, and so with the many existential and spiritual questions that arise as a consequence. If we are to be integrated practitioners, we need to have a handle on these too.

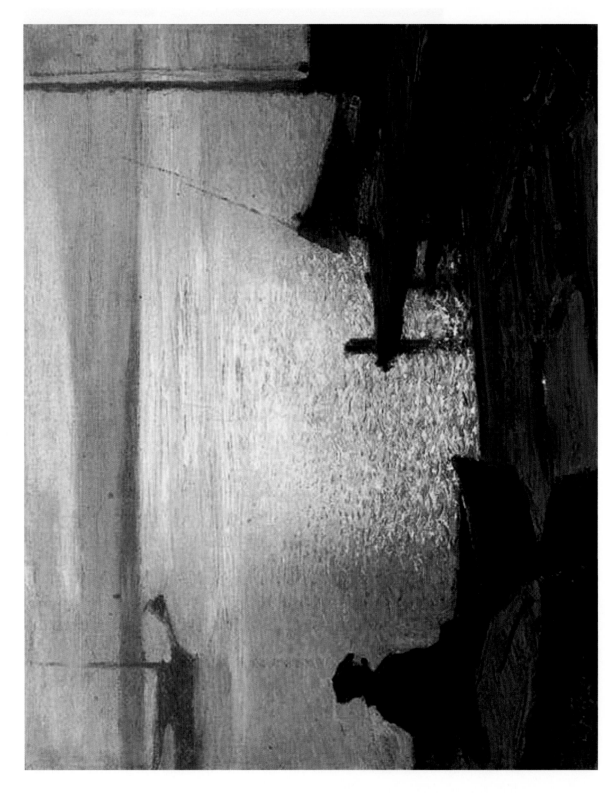

'*Along the Mystic River*' – for some reason I have found myself drawn to rivers as I have written this book, so a few will be popping up as we go along.[2]

So, in these workbooks we will try to look around the edges and to peer through the gaps, asking not just: 'What should we do?' but also 'Why should we do it?' and 'What does it all mean anyway?'

Finally, we don't have to practise long to realise that there are some things that make no sense, and from which no sense can be made. Random and chaotic events, reactions and emotions may arise, surprisingly. These can be both deeply troubling but also deeply wonderful, in that they can give expression to the inexpressible. We practitioners are practical people. We like to 'do' things. But sometimes there is nothing we can do, because there is nothing to be done. At these times, we have to just 'be'. For just 'being', for making sense of nonsense, and for making nonsense of sense, there is nothing better than poetry. So we will be seeing a fair bit of that too.

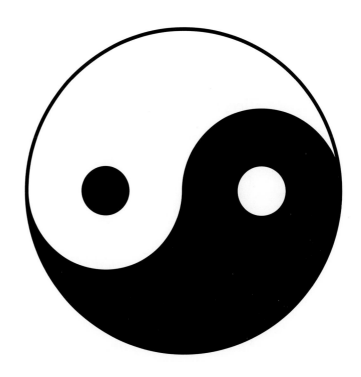

Symbols and rituals are fascinating things that in some way speak to us at a 'level beyond'. It is not often easy to make sense of them, and yet we may be surprised to find that our practice is full of them.

Ars Poetica

A poem should be palpable and mute
As a globed fruit,
Dumb
As old medallions to the thumb,
Silent as the sleeve-worn stone
Of casement ledges where the moss has grow –
A poem should be wordless
As the flight of birds.
*

A poem should be motionless in time
As the moon climbs,
Leaving, as the moon releases
Twig by twig the night-entangled trees,
Leaving, as the moon behind the winter leaves.
Memory by memory the mind–
A poem should be motionless in time
As the moon climbs.
*

A poem should be equal to:
Not true.
For all the history of grief
An empty doorway and a maple leaf.
For love
The leaning grasses and two lights above the sea–
A poem should not mean
But be.

– Archibald MacLeish[3]

POINTS AND PRIZES: SOMETHING FOR NOTHING

In the initial stages of this book, my publisher explained that medical publishing is at a turning point. Whereas before practitioners might choose a book that they would enjoy reading, nowadays they are too busy for that. So the upshot is that we only read books we need to read, rather than those we want to read.

A bit like Nanny McPhee . . .

The good news about adopting an integrated approach is we don't need to judge, we just need to adapt. If that is the way of the world, so be it, and so we have.

The particular way of the current world of health practice (at least where I currently work in the UK) appears to be a focus on objectives, outcomes, points and prizes. So the initial book has been adapted to match. Each chapter will contain activities and reflections that will meet common curriculum areas for medical and nursing practice. At the end of each book is a link to the Radcliffe Continuing Professional Development site, www.radcliffehealth.com/cpd, where you can download certificates that you can use for your CPD, appraisal or revalidation requirements.

OK, I admit it's a bit tongue in cheek, but there's no rule to say that we can't have fun while toeing the line, is there?

PROVISOS

I am, at heart, a practitioner, and a general practitioner at that. That means I am a bit of a jack of all trades, but master of none. I am partial, biased and subjective. The book is intended for all health practitioners but, inevitably, and despite my best efforts, no doubt the 'male', 'medical' and 'Western' nature of my experiences and thoughts will peep through. I hope you feel able to forgive them and look past them.

Also, I can quite honestly say that there is nothing new in this book, and I doubt there is anything in it that you could not find better argued and more coherently evidenced in other places. There is some philosophy, science, spirituality, art and poetry, but I am not a philosopher, scientist, guru, artist or poet. I am a health practitioner who dabbles.

So I have referenced those sources I can remember and can find. Others may be lost in the mists. But I do not claim any of the basic ideas in this book as my own. I have simply looked at them from my personal perspective and tried to put them together in a way that I have found useful in my own practice and in my own teaching. I hope you can enjoy them, and that you will forgive the numerous mistakes and omissions that you will undoubtedly find.

Chapter 1

The universe

> ## Question to chew over
>
> What does it mean to you 'to exist'? In what ways are you separate and independent from everything else, and in what ways are you related to and part of everything else?

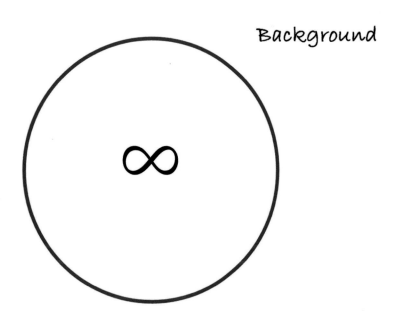

Background

As practitioners we like to be practical and focus on the specifics. But sometimes it is also good to reflect, and to consider everything (and nothing).

INTRODUCTION TO BOOK 5

In this book, we can change gear, and change focus a little. The previous four books have been practical in nature, which is reasonable given they are aimed at practitioners. But sometimes we practitioners like a bit of theory, and some time to stretch our minds beyond the confines of our day-to-day work.

This book aims to scratch that itch, by exploring some of the philosophy and science behind the concept of integrated practice. In line with the different tone of this book, we won't have 'activities' to complete, but rather 'questions to chew over'. Or not, as the mood takes you.

In some ways therefore this is an optional book, but it is included in the hope that some readers will find it satisfying.

INTEGRATION

In our exploration of integrated practice, and given that the last four books have been particularly focused on the 'practice', perhaps a good place to start is with the concept: 'integrated'.

What do we mean by integrated? Who is integrated with what? How?

Let's start at the beginning. One thing that everything in the universe shares is the state of existence.

When we say we exist, we mean that we 'stand out' within the universe, yet also belong as an integral part of the universe, while the universe is also an integral part of us. To understand what it is to be a 'healthy' human, and what it is to be 'integrated' within the universe, we therefore may find it useful to understand a little about the universe.

THE UNIVERSE

The universe seems to be an infinitely complex yet integrated, absolutely relational entity. The universe is the integrated relationship between space, time, energy, matter and forces. Even space and time, which to us seem to be fixed and static entities, seem to be relational. Within the relationship called 'special relativity',[4] space 'contracts' as time 'dilates', and vice versa.

This throws up quite a bizarre phenomenon. The faster we travel relative to another entity, the slower time passes; and vice versa. This is barely observable at the relative speeds we travel as humans, but is noticeable at the cosmic level.

The universe 'contains' all matter and energy, which are also relational (the concept of mass–energy equivalence, which derives from the first law of thermodynamics). As matter increases in speed, it gathers more energy. Einstein showed that nothing can travel faster than the speed of light. The reason for this is the equivalence of matter and energy.

As an object goes faster (gaining more energy) it also gains more mass. As the ratio between mass and energy is the speed of light, the closer to the speed of light

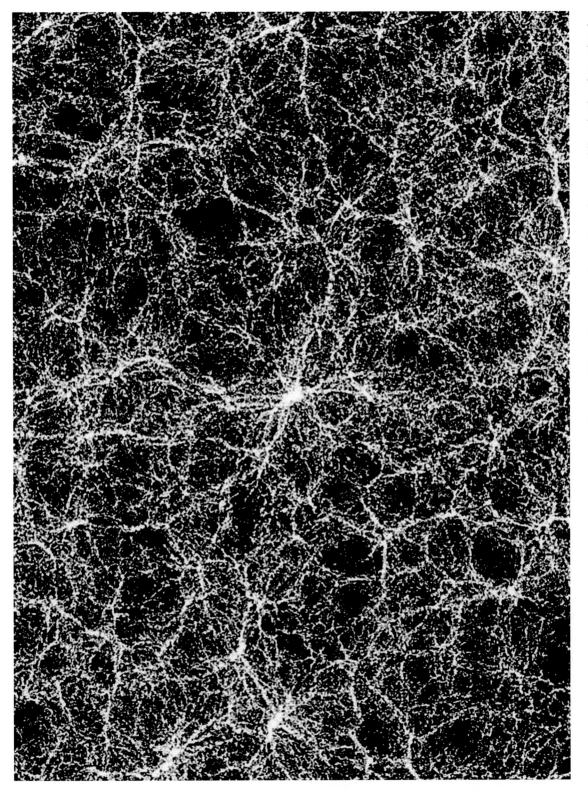

The fundamental interconnectedness and interrelatedness of the universe.[5] Note how it looks like a rather chaotic three-dimensional 'foam' rather than ordered and geometric.

an object travels, the more massive it becomes. The increase is without limit and becomes infinite at the speed of light. To move an infinitely massive object would require an infinitely massive amount of energy, which there isn't.

String theory suggests that relationality exists right down to the level of basic forces and matter. It suggests that all energy and matter may derive from relationships between one-dimensional oscillating 'strings'. These are thought to be of two kinds: closed loops which create 'gravitons' (the elementary particle of gravity), and open loops which create photons (the elementary particle for electromagnetic force and electromagnetic energy).

EXISTENCE

While all of this may be quite difficult to comprehend, we can probably at least all agree that we 'exist' in some form or another, or we wouldn't be having this conversation right now. However, existence is fundamentally tied up with the universe. We exist as part of the universe, and the universe exists within us.

So we cannot really say anything about what is *not* the universe, except that it is 'no-thing'. By definition we can have no experience or understanding of no-thing, so it is a mystery to us. But, there is one thing we can say something about, and that is we are somehow in relationship with it. Every-thing (the universe) is in a state of relationship with no-thing (not the universe). One is defined by not being the other.

So what is 'existence? Complexes or 'states' of matter and energy 'ex-ist' (stand out) with varying degrees of complexity (entropy[6]) within the continuum of space and time against a background of the nothingness, which is nothing. So 'existence' appears to be a relational 'standing out' of 'things 'against the 'background' of 'non-existence'.

As conscious beings, we are aware that we ourselves ex-ist (stand out) against the background of the rest of the universe. We have a sense of being individual, contained and self-governing; and in some ways we are. But we may also lose sight of the fact that we are also a small, relational part of a broader, universal relational whole.

> A human being is part of the whole called by us universe, a part limited in time and space. We experience ourselves, our thoughts and feelings as something separate from the rest: a kind of optical delusion of consciousness. This delusion is a kind of prison for us, restricting us to our personal desires and to affection for a few persons nearest to us. Our task must be to free ourselves from the prison by widening our circle of compassion to embrace all living creatures and the whole of nature in its beauty. The true value of a human being is determined by the measure and the sense in which they have obtained liberation from the self. We shall require a substantially new manner of thinking if humanity is to survive.
>
> – Albert Einstein, 1954

RELATIONAL AND BALANCED CREATIVITY WITHIN THE UNIVERSE

Relationality within the universe is fundamentally creative, in that each level of relationality creates a total that is bigger the sum of its parts. For example, relationality between atoms creates molecules, between molecules creates cells, between cells creates sentient beings, between sentient beings creates ideas, and between ideas creates societies and cultures.

There is a name for entities which are reducible, but within which each 'whole' level is greater than the sum of the parts. That name is 'holon'.[7]

This moment, this love, comes to rest in me
many beings in one being
In one wheat grain a thousand sheep stacks

Inside the needle's eye
a turning night of stars

There is a light seed grain inside
you fill it with yourself or it dies

I am caught in this curling energy, your hair
who ever is calm and sensible
is insane!

— Rumi

The relationships between the entities of the universe are balanced in many different ways, and at many different levels. There are balanced relationships between oscillations in strings, between forces, between matter and energy, between subatomic particles, between atoms, between molecules, between organic and non-organic entities, between cells, between organisms, between physiological systems, between people, between cultures, between societies, biological and ecological systems, between planets and stars, and between galaxies.

So relationality and balance seem to be integrally part of everything within the universe.

As sentient beings, we are aware of many of these balances, and unbalances. We are unusual compared to most entities in the universe in that we are sentient, which means that that we can experience these balances and unbalances as a sense of pleasure or of displeasure. When the balances are pleasing to us, often when they obey mathematical or musical patterns, they are called 'harmonic'. We can experience harmonies with all our five senses, such as restful music, the scent of a summer garden, the taste of a good meal, the pleasing touch of massage, or the aesthetic beauty of perfect form.

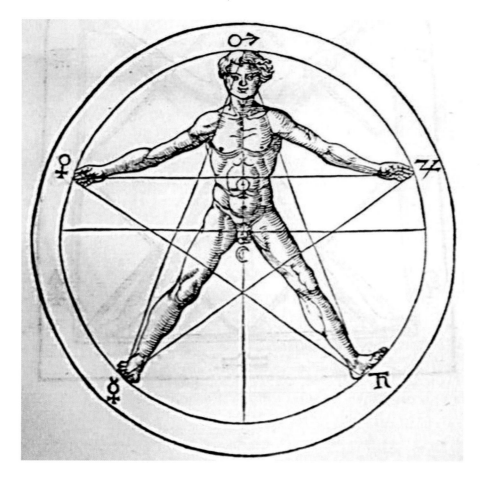

Golden ratio.[8] Diagrams of 'perfect man' incorporating pentagrams demonstrate the golden ratio (this one from Agrippa's 'Libri Tes de Occulta Philosophia'). Note the human addition of geometric shapes. We will come back to this.

As sentient human beings; and (as far as we are yet aware) the most highly developed of all universal complex entities, we are the crowning achievement of the integrated, harmonically balanced, relational creativity of the universe.

> In physical terms, we have a very, very low entropy. From the second law of thermodynamics (that entropy of a system always increases or stays constant) that also means we can become very easily unbalanced, discordant and disintegrated.

As health practitioners, it may therefore be worth considering that one of our prime aims is to help our patients achieve and maintain the highest state of integrated, harmonically balanced relationality as possible.

This is an idea we would like to play with a little more, and so the creation of integration, balance and harmony are the main themes of these workbooks.

To see a world in a grain of sand,
And a heaven in a wild flower,
Hold infinity in the palm of your hand,
And eternity in an hour.

– William Blake (from 'Auguries of Innocence')

Question to chew over

In your life, and in the lives of your patients, what entities can become dis-integrated and unbalanced, and what can you do to try to reintegrate and rebalance them?

Chapter 2

Time

Question to chew over

In your practice, in what ways does time govern you and in what ways do you govern time?

SPACE–TIME EVENTS

From our human perspective, time seems to flow from past, to present, to future. However, from both scientific and philosophical perspectives, this is not at all obvious, or indeed true.

As mentioned in the last chapter, within the space–time continuum, scientists suggest that time is relative to the speed and positions of the observers (with time running 'slower' for a person travelling faster relative to a companion).

It is very difficult to get one's head around the apparent difference between how we experience time and how science says time is. Scientific laws of the universe are time symmetric, which means that they allow for time to 'flow' in both directions (past to future as well as future to past). Indeed, some physicists speculate the universe may reverse direction and start moving back to low entropy again, therefore 'reversing' our experience of time.

What science seems to tell us is that there are 'events' and that these events happen in the continuum of time and space. Each event therefore has four coordinates: time and the three coordinates of space, which are length, width and depth. Space–time events do not flow; they just are.

It helps to compare our conception of time to our conception of space, which we do not experience as a flow. We can understand and accept that 'here', 'there' and 'somewhere else' are relational concepts that do not flow from one to another. Indeed, we can easily understand and accept these terms have no meaning if we take away the perspectives of the observers from whom they are near, far or over there. For observers in different places, far for me may be near for him; and vice versa.

In the same way, in order for time to 'flow', it needs someone to observe it, and experience things having happened, things happening and things that will happen. The fact that we cannot experience states that have not happened, but we can remember things that have happened, gives us the sense that things flow through time.

According to science, the only thing that seems to 'flow' in the universe is entropy, with the universe apparently moving from a low entropy (organised) state to a high entropy (disorganised) one. This is easier to understand. We all can imagine cold milk and hot black coffee mixing to form brown moderately cool coffee, but we can't imagine warm brown coffee separating into hot black coffee and cold milk. How on earth the universe came to be a highly organised entity is anyone's guess![9]

In summary, then, what we can say is that there are space–time 'events' happening in the continuum of time and space. Therefore all 'events' have four coordinates: time, and the three coordinates of space (length, width and depth). These space–time events do not 'flow', they just 'are'.

The essence of 'now-ness' runs like fire along the fuse of time.

– George Santayana

THE EXPERIENCE OF THINGS 'FLOWING'

So how do we explain the very clear experience that we have of time 'flowing'?

As we mentioned above, the answer seems to rest upon the position and attributes of the person who does the observing. For anything to appear to 'flow' within the universe, either within space or within time, it 'needs' someone to *observe* it flow. Without an observer, flow does not happen.

This is again a very difficult idea to grasp. After all, we can imagine rivers flowing while we are asleep, irrespective of the fact we are not currently observing them. But the key to this apparent mystery is the word 'imagine'. The flowing still continues, because we still keep observing, only in our imagination rather than by direct observation.

Any 'observer' of flow must have these crucial attributes.

- Consciousness: she must be able to observe and be conscious of the event not having happened yet (what we call the future), the event happening (what we call the present) and the event having happened (what we call the past).
- Memory: she must be able to link these events together into a chain in her own memory.

Without consciousness and memory, there is no 'flow'. In other words, our sense of time flowing is really a creation of our consciousness in combination with our memory.

We will go over this in more detail later on, but through our sensory and neurological apparatus our consciousness receives new sensory information about the current state of the matter, forces and energy of the 'external' universe, and new sensory information helps generate new 'internal' brain states. However, consciousness also assists in the further evolution of new brain states, by recalling previous brain states and anticipating future brain states. This creates the sense that we are moving from past to present to future. Thus, even though time does not flow in practice, our perception and memory of a relational sequence of events certainly gives us the perception of time flowing.

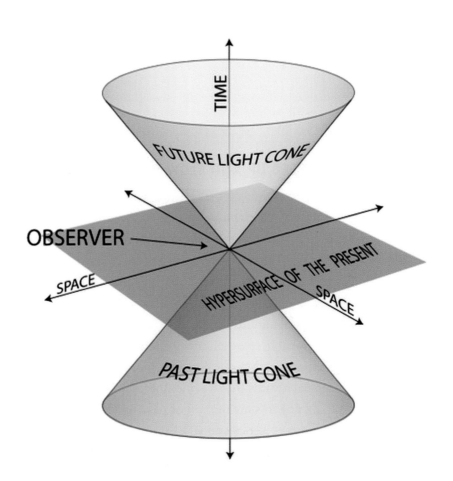

Three-dimensional space–time in a 2-D picture.[10] Note the relationship between time, space and energy, creating space–time 'moments'.

The fascinating diagram shown above[11] shows three-dimensional space–time in a 2-D picture. The place where the two cones of light 'intersect' is the space–time 'event' or the 'moment'. When a space–time event happens, light from the event spreads out at light speed, travelling in all directions, within space (horizontal plane) and time (vertical plane). In the 'past' light travels in 'towards' the event, narrowing down until it meets the actual event (in the present) and then spreads out again (in the 'future').

Note that the event's 'present' is a relative concept different for observers in relative motion. A different observer will see the event in a different place in space **and** in time.

So, for an 'event' to be perceived requires a conscious observer.

If we could draw a picture of what actually happens in the multidimensional universe of practice, this would take place in four dimensions, so that, instead of a cone, light would form spheres 'coming out' of the page on all sides of it. Past light would be a contracting sphere and future light an expanding sphere, with both converging to a point at the exact time/space coordinates of the event.

> *Thy letters have transported me beyond*
> *This ignorant present, and I feel now*
> *The future in the instant*
>
> — *Macbeth* (Shakespeare)

CAN TIME REALLY SPEED UP AND SLOW DOWN?

It is all very well saying that time can speed up and slow down. But if we can only really experience this by travelling through space at extraordinary speeds, it is stretching it a bit to say that it is of any relevance to us, as simple health practitioners, travelling through practice (pretty slowly . . .).

But just hold on a minute.

Speaking of which: are you really going to hold on for a complete minute or just pause briefly, interpreting 'a minute' relatively, as a pause of unquantifiable duration?

You see, in fact we are able to experience time going faster, slower, stopping and even reversing all the time: within our consciousness. We can leap forward into an imagined future, leap backwards into a remembered past, and have the experience of time standing still, going in slow motion or passing very quickly. In our thoughts or dreams, we can compress weeks and years into moments.

But hold on a second. Surely that's cheating. What goes on in our consciousness isn't the same thing at all as what goes on in the real world?

Really? What is the 'real world' and what is 'consciousness', if not the 'real world'? Aren't they the same thing? We never experience the real world except through consciousness, and we never experience consciousness outside the real world.

But we will come to that later. For now, please read on.

OUR CONCEPTIONS AND PERCEPTIONS OF TIME

This is all rather mind-boggling, so let's take stock, and find our bearings.

Even if we cannot pin down exactly what time is, or how it might (or might not) 'flow', we can at least be fairly confident about a few things. For humans like us, with consciousnesses and memories like us, whatever time does or doesn't do . . .

- We still perceive it as moving from past, to present and to future. So, practically speaking, it doesn't really matter whether this is actually due to the flow of entropy or an inherent property of time.
- Our conception of the present is creative, in that we take external sense data and abstract that into a world of self-created entities like thoughts, ideas and memories. So we 'create' our own experience of existence within our consciousness.
- Our conception of the past is creative, in that we store and our consciousness recalls memories of previous actions; these appear to us to follow a linear chain of memories (even if these memories are based upon a false perception of time).
- Our conception of future is creative, in that we have never experienced it, and so can have no 'memory' of actions not yet taken. So the future is, at least to our conception, a blank canvas upon which our consciousness can create and paint many different possible future scenarios.
- We seem, from a conceptual point of view, to have some freedom (although far from unlimited) to act in various ways at any one time, and each of the actions will lead to a different chain of events. We therefore have a conception of ourselves as being at least partly self-governing (autonomous) and self-creating.

As our 'past', 'present' and 'future' are all self-created conceptions; and as we have at least some degree of choice over which actions we take at any particular 'present', **we can quite literally say we create our own existence: past, present and future**.

Furthermore, these three concepts all depend on each other. We can have no past without 'presents' that have occurred; and we can have no 'future' without continuing to act in the 'present'. Therefore, not only is time apparently relational from a scientific point of view, it is certainly also relational from a conceptual point of view.

As practitioners, our ability to be able to 'create' our own present, and therefore our own futures, is absolutely crucial, for it is by helping our patients 'create' more healthy presents that we help them create more healthy futures. For this reason we will be experimenting with the practical implications of 'creativity' in health practice through the rest of this book.

An Exchange of Gifts

As long as you read this poem
I will be writing it.
I am writing it here and now
before your eyes,
although you can't see me.
Perhaps you'll dismiss this
as a verbal trick,
the joke is you're wrong;
the real trick
is your pretending
this is something
fixed and solid,
external to us both.
I tell you better:
I will keep on writing this poem for you
even after I'm dead.

– Alden Nowlan[12]

Question to chew over

Look at your practice in the past, present and future. What are you creating in each?

Chapter 3
The 'self'

In the last chapter we saw that those things we think of as being concrete and foundational – space and time – are not quite as concrete as we might have thought, or liked. In this chapter we will (nervously) consider what this means for us, as human beings.

Health practice is fundamentally a practice between 'selves' – the practitioner (myself), the patient (yourself) and the many other people that are involved in any process of health practice (themselves). We might therefore think that a clear concept of 'selfhood' should be central to an understanding of health practice.

We use words like 'identity' or 'self' to account for the fact we 'feel' the same over time and over experience. But we know we are not physically identical over time. Our bodies are dynamic and constantly changing.

If we feel identical, but we know we are not physically identical, what does that mean? Can we pin down exactly what a 'self' is, and what it is not? When we look at this question we find that it is not at all easy, and in fact that philosophers have been wrestling with this question for thousands of years. Here is a quick summary of the main streams of thought on the conundrum of personal identity.

Perhaps our sense of identity is not to do with the 'body' but something else, maybe the 'mind'. If that were to be true, we would have to assume that 'mind' is somehow fundamentally different to 'body'. But this is a highly problematic assumption. We know our mind seems to be intimately related to brain function, and the brain is physical. If we change the way our brain functions, we change the way our mind functions.

Maybe the self is the relation between 'body' and 'soul'. But this assumption is again highly problematic. We have to answer the question: what is 'soul'? Why can't we see it? We might answer we can't see it because it is of another 'substance' that is wholly different to the physical substances of the universe, and therefore unseeable and unknowable. But if so, we would then have to answer another extremely difficult question: how do two substances of completely different nature communicate with each other? We would need to postulate a new 'third substance' to act as a communicator, but that just takes us back to the beginning, only now with three 'substances' to explain rather than two.

Maybe our identity as a 'self' is something to do with 'consciousness'.[13] This seems at face value to be useful, but leaves some questions unanswered. For example, does this mean we stop being ourselves when we are asleep or unconscious? In any case, this solution is not really a solution at all. To explain one tricky entity (the self) we have postulated another equally tricky one: consciousness. This solution therefore solves one problem only by creating another. What is consciousness?

OK, let's push on. Perhaps it is to do with consciousness, only maybe there is no 'single' consciousness, rather 'bundles' of perceptions which are constantly changing and evolving, but which are linked by sense and memory.[14] This solution seems a good one, at face value, but on closer inspection we find that it also begs a question. This time we have created another entity: 'perception'. To 'whom' do these perceptions belong? And, again, how do the 'bundles' of perception relate to the physical 'matter' of our bodies?

Different philosophers have chosen to get off this never-ending train of thought at different stations. None seems to have got to the end of the line and arrived at a wholly satisfactory conclusion. It seems that none of us really knows the answer, so all that is left to us is belief. We may believe one or more of the solutions suggested above, or something else entirely.

However, for the sake of this book, please consider another solution. Perhaps the only rational answer to these infinitely regressing and circular questions is that in fact there is no self at all. Perhaps selfhood is just an illusion created by our awareness of our own awareness. In other words, it is a verb with no subject or object. There is no one being aware, and no one who is being the subject of awareness.

There is just 'being aware', which is a function of the way our bodies and brains works together.[15]

THE SELF AS RELATIONAL, INTEGRATED AND COMPLEX

Let's go back a bit. Let's try to find some points of agreement.

A useful place to start our exploration of this fascinating subject might be to set out those things that we can probably agree on, such as the following.

● As readers of this book, we are all 'selves' and we all 'exist'.

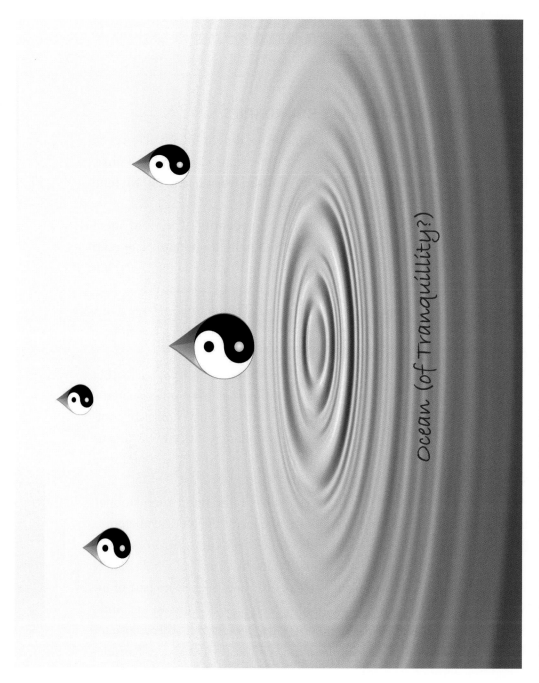

Ocean (of Tranquillity?)

Just like raindrops, we seem to have an individual existence, albeit very briefly, but we also seem to be integrally part of a much broader universal system, from which we originate and to which we return

- We exist as an integral part of the universe, and the universe is an integral part of us.
- We are highly complex, integrated, relational beings.
- We are made up of highly complex and relational parts (e.g. molecules, cells, organs and systems) which have an existence in their own right.
- We form part of even more complex and relational wholes (e.g. families, cultures, societies, the biosphere and the noosphere[16]) which also have an existence in their own right.

THE PROBLEM OF BLURRY AND LEAKY BOUNDARIES

These statements seem very plausible, and difficult to disagree with. However, although we may accept, and even 'know', that we are complex, relational beings, usually it doesn't 'feel' that way. If we think about our own existence at all, we tend to think of ourselves as whole, individual and concrete.

In philosophy, this is sometimes referred to as having 'identity'. The word 'identity', however, is clever, because it can capture both our plurality (identity can refer to the set of characteristics by which we are known and recognisable to others) but also our singularity (identity also refers to the quality of being the same).

As we have seen, the word 'exist' means to 'stand out'. That definition begs a very big question: stand out from what? In order for us to 'stand out' there has to be a background against and from which we can stand out.

If we think about it, this becomes tricky. We know we stand out from each other and from other entities both in a material way (standing out from other material entities) and also in a psychological way (standing out from other psychological entities). However, when we start trying to grope for the boundaries of these 'existences' we find it is incredibly difficult to find an exact place where 'I' stop and something/ someone else starts.

Whichever perspective of myself that I choose to take, I find that I am relational: part of something bigger and made up of something smaller. At energetic, subatomic, atomic, cellular, familial, cultural, ecological and cosmic levels I am always one holon within a stack of smaller and greater holons, all within the universal whole. There is no part of me that did not come from somewhere else, and there is no part of me that will not end up somewhere else. I can lose bits of me, or add bits to me, and I will still feel me. I can fall asleep, become unconscious, become demented, lose my memories – and I will still, in some sense, be me. I am mostly just space. Particles can pass through me without meeting any other particle en route. When I think of my consciousness, I can see that many of my ideas came from others, as do my language, my beliefs, my ethics and my standards.

So it seems we do have boundaries, but they are leaky and blurry.

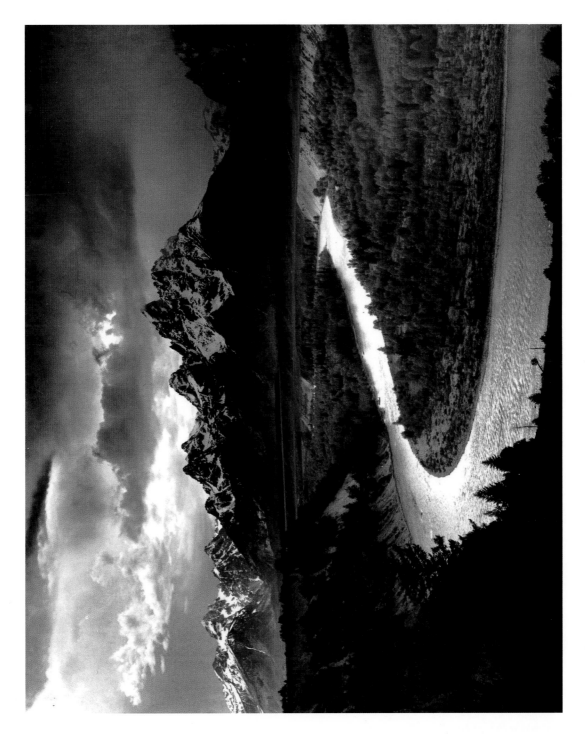

The 'river'[17] analogy may be helpful in understanding the 'both/and' nature of selfhood. A river is both one thing and also a constantly changing, utterly relational thing, which is never the same from one moment to the next. A spectrum is a particular dynamic perspective of a greater whole (being the part we can sense of a much broader relational and continuous whole).

SO WHO AM I?

The short and long answer to this question is, we both know and we don't know.

Each of us instinctively 'knows' who we are, because we live as ourselves every minute of every day. On the other hand, when we try to pin down what it is that is inherently and concretely 'me', we find we are like a set of smaller Russian dolls, within an even greater set of larger Russian dolls.

It is therefore difficult to escape the sense that, at some level, our sense of difference between 'me' and 'not me' is partly illusional, as we are connected to everything and everything is connected to us. The idea that our sense of selfhood may be partly illusional can be a profoundly disconcerting one, but it can also (potentially) be a profoundly liberating one, and one which opens up tremendous opportunities for health practice.

Game: Who am I?

This is an easy game to play, although difficult to finish. Just keep asking yourself and don't let yourself off the hook until you finish.

E.g. A conversation between two of my internal selves

Self 1: Who are we?
Self 2: We are a doctor, a man, we are English, and we are a father, etc.

Self 1: Those are categories not us. Which father, which man, which doctor are we?
Self 2: Well, we are the doctor that was born in London, that is the son of Tony and Rhian, whose families comes from Lincolnshire and Wales.

Self 1: Fine. So now we know where we come from and which categories we belong to, but you still haven't told us who we are!
Self 2: OK, OK! We are the London-born doctor/son of Tony and Rhian, who has five children and who is currently looking out of the window.

Self 1: No need to get snotty. How would I know you are not an identikit robot model of that Justin?
Self 2: Because I am inside our head, talking to us!

Self 1: So, we exist in our head?
Self 2: Well, yes, but it's what we do with our head that matters.

Self 1: So what do we do with our head?

Self 2: We take in data, we abstract a bit, we chuck in a few memories, we get haunted by all sorts of suppressed hidden stuff, we think about things, we make choices and then sometimes we do something?

Self 1: What kind of things do we do?
Self 2: We do the things that we want to do.

Self 1: What sort of things do we want to do?
Self 2: We do the kind of things that are important to us.

Self 1: What, like gazing out of the window?
Self 2: Well, yes, but other stuff too. We do things that we are driven to do, by our instincts, by our thoughts, by our morals.

Self 1: So you are saying we are what we do?
Self 2: Yes, I suppose so.

Self 1: What, like gazing out of the window?
Self 2: Well, OK, maybe not the automatic actions. It may be better to say that we exist (in the eyes of ourselves and others) in the choices that we make that make us stand out from everyone else.

Self 2: But who makes those choices?
Self 3: Shut up! I'm trying to get some sleep!

THE IMPORTANCE OF MEMORY

One of the reasons we have such a strong sense of personal 'identity' is because we can remember being the same person since . . . well, as long as we can remember. We each have a very strong sense of continuity with ourselves in both the past and future. From our human perspective, time seems to flow, from past, to present, to future. But as we have seen, time does not 'flow' any more than space does. It is just part of the fabric of the universe. Concepts such as 'past' and 'future' don't really have much scientific meaning. There are just 'events' in space–time.

Nevertheless, our memories exist, we do have a clear sense of chronological 'flow' of time, and we have created machines (clocks) which clearly move according to our sense of this flow. Therefore, we cannot simply ignore the problem.

One way to consider the relationship between memory and identity is to take a 'biological' approach and suggest that in fact there is an identity of biological *processes* over time even if there is no identity of biological ingredients and constructs. While the parts may change, each biological state we take as humans is built upon previous biological states. This is difficult to dispute, but again does not really deal with the sense of 'self' – it just skirts around it, by making 'selfhood' a product of biological processes. So in fact the process-identity model is really a hidden 'no-self' model in disguise.

Another way to consider the relationship between memory and identity is to take a 'psychological' approach and suggest we have continuity of mind. In this construction we create different 'mind states' and link these together through memory. Memory retains many of the events that have taken place in our existence, and places these in a chronological sequence, which gives us our sense of 'psychological continuity'.

Unfortunately, again, on closer inspection this approach is also problematic. For a start, we don't have true psychological continuity through memory. There are many mind states we do not remember. We do not usually remember much about our sleep, nothing about being anaesthetised, and very little about early childhood or our time in the uterus. Despite that, most of us feel we do not 'stop' being 'ourselves' in any of these states.

Furthermore, this is also a rather cunningly disguised no-self model. It postulates a new entity (mind) to explain the one we are puzzled about (identity). We can't locate mind any more easily that we can locate consciousness, perception or soul.

So, while we are all pretty clear that memory is important in helping us develop a sense of identity, when we try to pin it down, we find everything gently evaporates, leaving us with only ephemeral concepts and creations, and no concrete self or identity at all.

WHY IS ALL THIS IMPORTANT TO HEALTH PRACTICE?

While some of this discussion may seem like idle and fruitless speculation, it is difficult to avoid the nagging feeling that it is actually quite important to health practice.

After all, as health practitioners we are 'selves' trying to help other 'selves'. So a sense of what that selfhood means is presumably quite important. Furthermore, health has something to do with 'whole-ness' (and indeed the two words have the same origin). So a sense of what it is to be whole, less than whole, and more than whole is presumably quite important too.

Finally, everything that happens between the practitioner and patient happens within the context of the relationship between practitioner and patient. So a sense of our own relationality, the relationality of our patients, and the relationality between those two relationalities is presumably quite important as well!

We have very good reasons to want this problem to go away: we are really very busy, we are practical people and we want to get on. But we have a name for people who cling to irrationally held beliefs in order to explain their existences. And we tend to put them on medication.

So, if we are to be consistent, we either have to start questioning our most deeply held and cherished beliefs, or we have to accept our own diagnostic categories might apply to ourselves as much as to our patients.[18]

It is as though you have an eye
That sees all forms
But does not see itself.
This is how your mind is.
Its light penetrates everywhere
And engulfs everything,
So why does it not know itself?

– Foyan

Question to chew over

To what extent do you know yourself and to what extent are you a mystery to yourself? How might this impact on how you practice, or indeed on how you exist?

Chapter 4

Consciousness

Question to chew over

What are you conscious of? What creates your consciousness?

Can anything be said to 'exist' outside the medium of your consciousness? If so: what and how?

WHAT IS CONSCIOUSNESS?

We briefly touched on consciousness in the last chapter on 'self', and many of the themes are similar. However, being conscious is a particular state of being a 'self', and it relates very strongly to our state of health which is, to a great extent, a state of consciousness.

So selfhood and consciousness seem to be interrelated in a circular way. Given that we can't easily define selfhood, it should be of no surprise to discover that consciousness is similarly difficult to define. Consciousness and awareness are similar, but they are not the same. We can be aware of things we are not conscious of, and we can be conscious of things we are not aware of. Consciousness seems to be something to do with ideas, representations, beliefs, attitudes and motivations. It is also used in a psychoanalytical context to describe those drives and motivations that we are aware of.

So consciousness seems only to be defined by and with consciousness. Consciousness is what it is to be conscious, and that's clearly a bit circular . . .

I know what I know and that what I know is knowledge.[19]

NOUN-VERBS

Although we cannot define objectively what consciousness is, we can at least describe it subjectively, because we all have the personal experience of what it is to be conscious.[20]

We each have a sense of possessing a single and unified consciousness, but when we look a little more deeply, we find that consciousness seems to be multi-layered, relational and highly complex.

When we try to describe our consciousness, we always tend to describe it 'as' something, as if it were a noun. In order to describe anything 'as' something, we need both a subject (the person who does the describing), an object (the thing being described), and an action (the describing). In the case of consciousness, we find that consciousness is the subject *and* the object *and* the verb *all at the same time*.

This is an extremely strange and unsettling phenomenon, which does not really occur anywhere else in our experience.

For this extremely strange phenomenon, we need an extremely strange tool: a 'noun-verb'. But sadly we don't have that, so we will have to continue to wrestle with inadequate language.

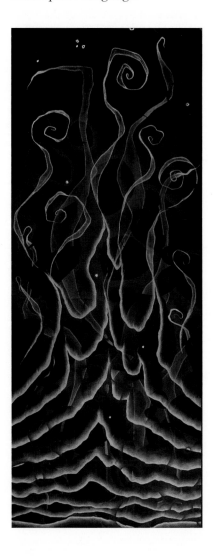

'Midnight Zen' – by Amandda Tirey Graham,[21] I have chosen this painting as it seems to capture the relational nature of consciousness, standing out (existing) against a background of something and nothing, building into ever more complex and abstract and freeform levels until eventually becoming one again with the nothingness.

'The evolution of the capacity to simulate seems to have culminated in subjective consciousness. Why this should have happened is, to me, the most profound mystery facing modern biology.'

– Richard Dawkins (1989)

PHILOSOPHICAL PERSPECTIVES OF CONSCIOUSNESS

The philosophy of consciousness starts (and ends) with an apparently insurmountable problem: consciousness is almost impossible to define. Generally, it seems to be something to do with having perceptions, thoughts or feelings. It is also something to do with being aware. Because it is indefinable, many philosophers think nothing sensible can be said about the subject, and go home.

> We have no idea how consciousness emerges from the physical activity of the brain and we do not know whether consciousness can emerge from non-biological systems, such as computers ... At this point the reader will expect to find a careful and precise definition of consciousness. You will be disappointed.
>
> – Frackowiak *et al.* (2004)

It seems that, despite claiming to be conscious, none of us really knows if consciousness is a genuine entity. Some doubt that it has any inherent reality at all. While we probably can agree that it is rare to find a conscious person who does not experience 'being conscious that they are conscious'; that is about the limit of what we can say with any certainty. After that we get stuck in a self-referential loop. The problem defining consciousness, and so the problems philosophically approaching consciousness, is that it is an inherently circular concept (I am aware that I am aware because I am aware of it).

The Nature of Consciousness

While we might have difficulty defining consciousness, we can at least say something about its nature. It seems that there may be many different levels of consciousness, rather than simply 'conscious' and 'unconscious'. However, if there is a spectrum of levels we can at least describe the two ends of the spectrum.[22]

- The awareness of simple sensory data (from sight, smell, touch, hearing etc.). Any things we pick up by sensory data are referred to as 'phenomena'. So we can call this phenomenal consciousness.
- The awareness of complex ideas, reasons, thinking, analysing, remembering and choosing. These are all 'concepts', so we can call this conceptual consciousness.

The suggestion that these are poles of a spectrum rather than separate entities comes from thinking about things like emotions, which seem to have elements of both sensory and conceptual awareness. When I get angry I get angry ideas and I get angry sensations. They are not separate.

Because of these two apparently different 'poles' of consciousness, the history of philosophy of consciousness has been particularly influenced by the question of whether consciousness is 'dualist' (i.e. made up of two separate, phenomenal and conceptual, entities) or 'monist' (i.e. one entity, of which different perspectives can be taken – phenomenal and conceptual) or multiple ('bundles' of many entities).

Descartes (in *The Description of the Human Body*, published in 1647) famously distinguished between two substances: mind and body. In so doing he lent his name to the 'Cartesian dualism' that dominated philosophy up until the post-modern era, and arguably still dominates medical thinking to this day. A dualist philosophy of mind and body has, however, been pretty well fatally undermined by the mind–body problem which is this: if the mind and body are of fundamentally different nature, how do they communicate with each other?

Dualistic interpretations seem increasingly difficult to maintain when it comes to consciousness. We can talk about the 'external world' (to describe the world of matter, forces, energy, space and time, which we can physically sense using our sensory apparatus) and the 'internal world' (to describe our world of concepts, ideas, beliefs and emotions). However, when it comes to consciousness, these classifications are inaccurate and misleading. We sense the world both 'inside' and 'outside' our physical boundary (our skins) through highly complex homeostatic, immunological and neurological systems, so sensing is not just a facet of the 'external world'. Similarly, our 'internal' conceptual world *is* the external world, or at least all we can know of it.

We are not able to intercept information signals along immunological or neurological pathways and analyse them as raw binary data (as we can, for example, in computers). The 'sensing' happens at the same instant as the 'conceptualising', in the same place (the brain) to the same person (me). Therefore, dualisms such as mind/body, internal/external, subject/object, and perception/conception are probably inherently misrepresentative and misleading.

The alternative to a 'dualist' philosophy of consciousness is the 'monist' approach, which suggests that mind and body are the same thing. Monist approaches can be divided broadly into physicalism (mind is just matter organised in a particular way), idealism (only thought truly exists whereas matter is simply an illusion created by thought) and neutral monism (mind and matter are aspects of a third entity that is neither of them).

In more recent times, philosophy and neuroscience have become closely intertwined, so it becomes hard to differentiate one from the other. These approaches are all forms of physical monism, which look to explain consciousness as the product of the physical properties of the body and in particular in the neural events that occur in the nervous system (e.g. Dennett 1993). Other philosophers and scientists have looked beyond classical physics to see if quantum physics can explain consciousness (*see* page 43).

Logically, though, the philosophical exploration of consciousness seems inescapably trapped in paradox. Consciousness becomes both the object of study and the subject doing the studying (not to mention the process by which we study). Without separation of subject and object (and indeed process) there can be no objective observation, no definition and no classification.

All we seem to be able to say is that consciousness seems to be another form of a 'holon', which is created by an increasingly complex relational interplay of many other complex, relational entities; and which itself can form part of ever greater holons (such as our families, our peer groups, our cultures and our societies).[23]

The Self-Creating Property of Consciousness

Perhaps even more important for health and health practice is the notion that our internal representations are self-created.

This is a very strange concept but one that is absolutely crucial to these workbooks.

To understand this we have to remember that whatever is going on 'out there', we can only ever experience 'in here', because all sensory data is immediately melded and interpreted by our internal conceptual apparatus through the medium of consciousness.

Furthermore, we have also to remember that we are subject, object and verb of our consciousness all at the same time.

When we look at the world around us, we see a wonderful world full of colours, people, landscapes, objects, textures and warmth. However, science tells us that all of these are simply relational combinations of forces, energy and matter. Things like colour, warmth and beauty do not have any existence in the physical world. They only exist because our consciousness creates them as we go along.

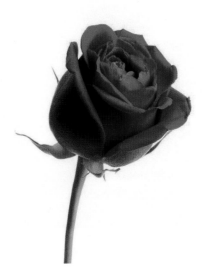

To get a feel for the mystery of self-creation, consider the following question: 'Is a rose red at night?'[24]

What we represent 'internally' is not the same as the 'external' phenomena (matters, forces and energies) that trigger these representations. What we are conscious of is the sense data interpreted, classified and accreted to other concepts, memories, emotions and experiences almost instantly. Our consciousness creates itself as it goes along.[25]

Therefore, we can quite literally say that we create our own present. Furthermore, because our 'future' and 'past' (as we saw in Chapter 2) are actually the connection of a succession of 'presents', each building on the previous, and linked by memory, we can quite literally say that we create our own pasts and futures too.

If we put all this together, **we can quite reasonably say that we create our own existence**.

And we don't mean that figuratively.

What we can say is that consciousness *seems* to involve a process of pulling together and processing information, which we may loosely describe as sensory data, memories, emotions, ideas, plans, values, beliefs. Everything we perceive through our senses is immediately transformed into concepts, and we have no choice about that. We can't choose to switch our consciousness off and experience matter, energy and forces in their raw form. We can only experience these 'raw materials' of

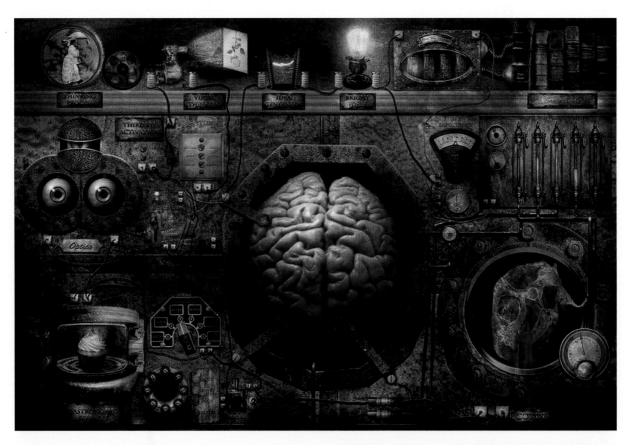

We are pretty sure consciousness has something to do with the interaction of the brain, the body and the environment. But no convincing scientific models yet exist ('Steampunk – Information Overload' by Mike Savad ©2012)[26]

existence with 'value added' – like colour, texture, depth and flow. That means we can't easily differentiate between the physical properties of the object of our observations and the concepts we layer onto our perceptions of those properties.

That's not to suggest that we create the basic building blocks of matter, energy and forces. We don't know how these were created, except to say that they appeared at the origin of the universe. But we can say we create everything else – our full experience of existence. From a practical perspective, our experience is the only experience of existence we have. We can only see through the eyes of our consciousness, and that consciousness creates itself. So it does not seem too much of a stretch to say that, in a practical sense at least, we create our own existences too.

SCIENTIFIC PERSPECTIVES OF CONSCIOUSNESS

As practitioners, we are scientists, so let's take a deeper scientific look at consciousness.

Science may never be able to discover or describe consciousness itself, because consciousness is an experience which has no observable physical existence, and is therefore closed to empirical enquiry. Fortunately, as practitioners, we don't need to get too bogged down with this. We are less interested in what consciousness is, and more interested in what consciousness *does*. Here the science is quite helpful.

Consciousness seems to function through the interplay in an infinitely complex array of continuous, self-referential loops. So we are not just conscious, we are also conscious of being conscious, and conscious of being conscious of being conscious (repeat ad infinitum).

These loops, somehow, enable us to experience, interpret and enrich our own existence. The loops seem to self-create, in the following, self-referential and circular process:

- We sense events going on around us in the 'external'[27] universe using our 'five senses' (*or however many we have*).
- We convert incoming sensory information into 'internal' representations within our consciousness (*whatever that is*).
- These 'internal' representations take the form of symbols (words and concepts) which we connect together with other symbols to create 'concepts' (*whatever those are*).
- We manipulate new and old concepts upon our internal representations like pieces on a chessboard, testing out combinations that may be effective in helping us reach our desired goal (*at last – we know what these are!*).
- We try these out by converting concepts to behaviours (*we know these too, although we may not always own up to them*).
- We sense the new events going on around us, represent these internally and decide if the behaviour was effective or not (*'effective'? Er, we're heading into the unknown again – see later*).
- We store the whole process in our memories (*don't even ask*) to give ourselves the

best chance of using effective and tested strategies and behaviours in the future (*which means what exactly?*).

Science, therefore, can be quite helpful in describing what consciousness does. We seem to be able to make some fairly confident suggestions that consciousness is produced by the interplay of many empirically observable factors. These include our physical bodies; the neurons and synapses of our nervous systems; our languages and symbols;[28] our families; or our societies. The reason we can make these assertions with some confidence is that we can observe them. For example, we know that brain damage (e.g. coma, disorientation) and chemicals (e.g. psychotropic drugs) can affect consciousness in different ways (e.g. by putting us to sleep, waking us up, making us lose our memories, altering our perceptions of time, vision and hearing). These observations suggest there is a strong connection between the brain and consciousness, even if we don't know what that is or how it may work.

We can also fairly confidently suggest that physical 'neural processing' (which can account for sensory data processing and to a large extent automated behaviours) and 'information processing' (which can account for ideas, thoughts, memories etc.) must somehow be both linked by and integrated by our consciousness. Similarly, the advances of computer programming and artificial intelligence, which ultimately derive from strings of 1s and 0s, have made it very clear how incredibly and increasingly complex forms can be created from simple building blocks by powerful information-processing abilities. However, it is important to note that no one has created a computer that is self-conscious in the way that 'we' are.

There are some interesting theories on how brains could generate consciousness. One is 'neural Darwinism'[29] which basically suggests that our brains trigger numerous ideas in response to changes in our sensory input, and these ideas somehow 'compete' subconsciously until 'better' (or more relevant) ones win out and make it to our consciousness, with which we make conscious choices, again based on Darwinist principles of 'selection of the fittest'. However, how this selection process might happen is far from clear.

Another interesting (though highly speculative) suggestion is thinking about whether the brain may act in some way as a quantum field/system. The universe is currently described by both classical and quantum theories, both of which stack up according to observational evidence, but which do not yet correlate with each other. In a mind-bogglingly difficult way, quantum theory seems to prove that matter can exist in both particle and wave states, both at one and the same time. The 'decision' about which state matter ultimately takes (when someone tries to observe it) is made by the very process of observation.

In other words, it appears that when we observe matter in its dual wave-particle form, it instantly 'collapses' into either a wave or particle according to the way be observe it. If we observe it with apparatus to look for particles, it behaves as a particle. If we observe it with apparatus that looks for waves, it acts as a wave. Until it

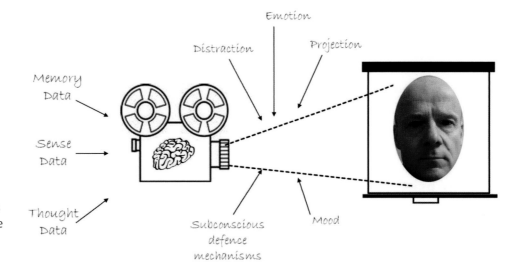

Memory Data

Sense Data

Thought Data

Distraction

Emotion

Projection

Subconscious defence mechanisms

Mood

We saw this image in workbook 4, but we'll use it again as it helps illustrate the self-creating nature of consciousness

is observed, it is not one or other, it is both. We can only state as a matter of prob-ability which (hence Einstein's famous – but later retracted – objection that 'God does not play dice').

Quantum mechanics seems, to me at any rate, completely bizarre, as it turns our world upside down. At quantum level at least, it suggests that observations are somehow in relationship with the thing which is observed, with each one influencing the other, in a kind of relational dance. This is a complete contradiction of the sub-ject–object dualism of our day-to-day experience, and it places into yet more serious doubt our ability to be objective about anything.[30]

On the other hand, this both/and duality of matter at quantum level is remarkably like our both/and experience of being conscious. Consciousness is *both* physical (in that it seems to derive from physical entities) *and* conceptual (in that it is a world of ideas and interpretations) at one and the same time. This also seems bizarre, although less obviously so. If we think about it, physical entities should behave according to predictable physical algorithms – like a computer. On the other hand, something that can be absolutely creative, generating new ideas wholly unrelated to the physical structures it derives from, should not behave according to physical algorithms. It would be like a computer creating and programming itself.

This is why some theorists have linked consciousness to both classical and quantum theories. From a 'classical' perspective, there appears to be a deterministic element to consciousness, because the brain behaves as a physical entity obeying classical physical theory to act in deterministic patterns. From a quantum perspect-ive, there appears to be a quantum element to consciousness, because the brain behaves as a quantum field which obeys quantum 'indeterminacy' and can 'collapse' as a matter of choice of the observer. As consciousness is both observer and observed (and also the act of observing) it could theoretically thus create itself.

David Bohm (1981)[31] and subsequently Roger Penrose (1989) drew on the parallels between philosophy of consciousness and quantum mechanics to try to find a deeper explanation. Bohm suggested that that there is a fundamental 'implicate' level to the universe, deeper than that we are currently aware of through science, and that all levels of 'explicate' existence, including consciousness, are based on that fundamental foundation. In other words he suggests that our phenomenal (physical) and conceptual (psychological) consciousness are both different perspectives of (and holons of) that fundamental implicate nature of the universe.

MYSTICAL PERSPECTIVES OF CONSCIOUSNESS

If this is beginning to sound to you more like religion than science, you are not alone. Religious and spiritual prophets and teachers have been claiming a deeper 'implicate' level to the universe for thousands of years.

These 'mystical' approaches arrive at a very similar place:[32] which is to say a sense of peaceful, creative interconnectedness and oneness with everything. Christian mysticism, Sufism in Islam, Jainism, Buddhism, and Vedanta Hinduism take this approach. Rather than trying to describe and explain how consciousness 'works' (a very Western, empirical and positivist stance) they simply try to explain how con-

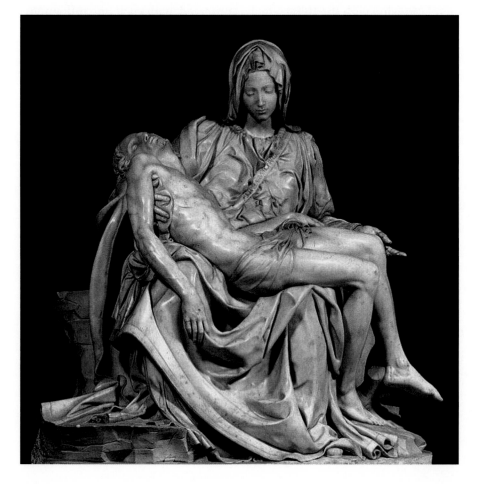

Consciousness integrates and creates. When you see this statue, what do you see? A disturbance in the time–space continuum? The interplay of force, energy and matter? A high entropy object? A lump of calcium carbonate? A piece of nonsense? A work of art? A sacred object? A historical artefact? All of those? Something else entirely?

sciousness 'is'. In other words, they describe and explore the *experience* of being conscious, at deeper and deeper levels of awareness.

The common aims of these mystical practices are to attain freedom from body–mind identification and to achieve release into absolute connectedness with the oneness of everything. By using meditative or deep mindfulness techniques, as well as other techniques such as rhythmical dancing, singing, starvation and psychedelic substances, mystics practise becoming more and more 'aware' of their own consciousness. This is a helical process of the watcher watching the watcher watching the watcher. At each stage, the watcher 'disengages' with that 'level' of consciousness, watching it rather than being it, and moving on to the next level.

To Buddhism, for example, oneness is interpreted as 'emptiness' (Dalai Lama 2010). Unlike nihilism, this is not a negative sense of emptiness. In emptiness one finds complete freedom from 'attachment' to the 'self'. Attachment to the self is a state of suffering, so becoming one with the emptiness is absolute release from suffering.

In some senses then, the scientific and mystical explorations of consciousness approach the same problem from different perspectives. Science tries to 'describe and explain' consciousness from an *external perspective* by looking for systems and ingredients which might explain 'how it works'. Mysticism tries to explain how it is to be conscious, and to describe the experience of being conscious, from an *internal perspective*. When mystics and scientists speak of consciousness as a single, unified expression of existence, deriving from matter and being at one with matter, from one perspective knowable and from another perspective unknowable, they almost seem to be speaking the same language.

Ultimately, though, perhaps consciousness is fundamentally unknowable because of its self-referential, self-defining, circular nature. We will look at these fundamental problems of knowledge in coming chapters. For now, though, it is not that either perspective (scientific, external or internal, mystical) is wrong. It may simply be that each is unprovable. If so, they are a matter of belief rather than of knowledge.

And we all believe something, even if that something is nothing.

SO WHAT DOES THIS ALL MEAN FOR HEALTH PRACTICE?

The long and the short of it is that we don't actually know what all of this means for health practice. The self-referential circularity of the logic and the science denies us any easy conclusions.

From one perspective, all of this may seem like idle and pointless speculation, but just hold on a minute. Surely this is all quite important for health practice? If we think a little, it does not take us long to create quite a long list of dualisms that we commonly fall into in health practice: body/mind, assessment/treatment, physician/surgeon, palliative/curative, emotional/behavioural, conventional/alternative, physical/psychological, and even healthy/unhealthy!

Given the apparent complex relationality of everything, perhaps we need to consider that these dualisms may not just be inaccurate, they may be seriously misleading and possibly undermining to our practice.

Dualisms give us comfort in a sea of uncertainty. They give a feeling of concreteness to otherwise nebulous concepts like health and healing. But in actual practice it is very difficult to separate out and draw boundaries between the 'subjective' world of concepts from the 'objective' world of senses. Everything we sense seems to be interpreted at some level, and our interpretations influence what and how we sense. Therefore our sense of being able to be objective and scientific observers of our patients and their 'health' may be fundamentally flawed.

And if that most basic premise is flawed, what does that mean for health practice?

If all we can say is that consciousness is something that creates itself, we are saying that we create ourselves and we co-create each other. This is a whole different kettle of fish. We might even go so far as to say it is an almost revolutionary concept for health practice.

'Self-creation' is probably not an idea we ever consider in our training or in our practice, but even brief contemplation shows how important it is. The way our patients perceive themselves, the way they perceive their health, the way we perceive them and their health, and the way they perceive us (and our health) will all be created, because we create ourselves, we co-create each other and we create everything around us.

It is therefore difficult to imagine we can master the art of health practice without mastering the art of self-creation and co-creation.

The implications of this are enormous.

old pond
a frog leaps in
water sound.

– Matsuo Basho: frog haiku[33]

Questions to chew over

In your concept of health, health practice, practitioners and patients, what are you creating? Do these creations have any concrete or independent 'existence' outside of consciousness? If so, what and how?

Chapter 5

Relationships

Question to chew over

How many different types of relationships can you have?

Relationships are relational entities too.

> No surprise there then...

This seems such a self-evident statement it hardly needs saying, let alone writing a whole chapter on. However, it is such a key topic that it deserves a little more exploration. After all, our relationship with our patients is possibly the fundamental relationship in our practice.

THE STRANGE DISAPPEARANCE OF YOU

In the last chapters, looking at the 'self' and 'consciousness', we came to a conclusion that, in a very real way, we 'create' our own present and therefore also 'create' our own pasts and futures too.

This is all well and good, but what happens when two or more people are in relationship? Who creates what in that situation?

Maybe we can backtrack a little. Traditionally, language allows us to have relationships in the first person (I and we), second person (you, both singular and plural) and third person (he/she/it and they/its). This is a useful categorisation for communication, but it may be actually a distortion of reality.

If we think about this a little more, can there ever be such a thing as a simple, independent 'you'. From your perspective, you are a 'me' not a 'you'. The only person for whom 'you' has any meaning is 'me'. And if 'I' am communicating with 'you', 'we' are already a 'we'. I start communicating with you as soon as I perceive you. I can never even think of you without creating you in my own consciousness, and what I create is my image of you coloured by my own consciousness. So I can never see 'you' entirely separately of 'me'. I only see 'we'.

The strange but apparently inescapable conclusion is that, as soon as I perceive you, or you perceive me, 'you' stop existing, and 'we' is created. As there cannot be a 'you' until I perceive you, that means that logically 'you' can never independently exist. You are always a 'me' or a 'we'.

THE 'BIG THREE' RELATIONSHIPS

So, while 'you' is a useful literary and descriptive device, in actual experience, it doesn't appear to actually exist. Instead, it appears that there are only three fundamental relationships: my relationship with myself (the 'me');[34] my relationship with you (the 'we'); and my/our relationship with other people or other things (the 'other'). These relationships are sometimes known as the 'big three'.[35]

At any moment of our existence, we are in one or more of these relationships. In fact it is impossible for us to exist outside at least one of these relationships. In a relational universe, everything can only ex-ist (stand out) in relation to something else.[36]

Before we move on, it is also helpful to consider what is not in these relationships: the 'other'. 'Other' is an extremely interesting concept. Without it, we can have no concept of 'self', because 'self' is by definition a separation from everything 'other'. Without the 'other' there could be no 'me' (Hegel). It doesn't just create our self-concept, it is essential in how we design and experience our self-concept. Without the 'other' to define ourselves against, who would we say we are? Our experience of existence is radically affected by the other. As soon as we become aware of another person or thing, we feel at once a sense of alienation and a desire to find a place relative to that other person or thing.

MANY ME'S

This relationality of our relationships takes an even stranger twist when we turn our focus onto ourselves. In fact the very phrase 'we turn our focus on ourselves' is a perfect example of the issue.

Who turns whose focus on whom?

It appears that, when we think about ourselves (*there you go again*) we set ourselves up as subject and object and verb. I am focusing. I am focusing on myself. And I am focusing with my consciousness which is conscious-ing.

He made that last one up.

Who are you to be talking about us like that?

Once we begin to see ourselves not as single, concrete unified selves but as relational, blurry and leaky selves, we can see that we 'contain' many different entities, each of whom has many different relationships and many different conversations.[37]

It may seem a bit odd to think of ourselves as being in relationship with ourselves, but of course we have conversations with ourselves all the time. We talk to ourselves, tell ourselves off, and try to calm ourselves down. We use what is called 'reflexive language', such as 'I spoke before I could stop myself', 'pull yourself together', or 'it seems ugly to me, but also beautiful in its own way'.

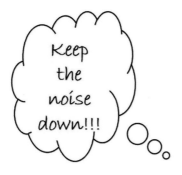

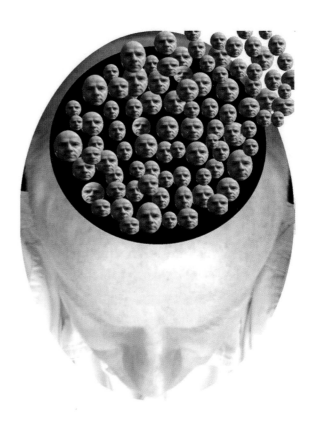

The strange phenomenon of many me's

Not only can we have conversations with ourselves, we can also be in many relationships with ourselves at one and the same time.

> We can be speaking to each other while enjoying the warm sun on our faces and listening to birdsong in the background while at the same time walking along the path and worrying about what we are going to cook for the kids for tea.

Food for thought

THE STRANGE (BUT VERY IMPORTANT) NOTION OF CO-CREATION

There is more . . .

We have already seen that each of us 'creates' our own reality through the inter-relationship of our existence within the universe and our consciousness of that existence (and the consciousness of the consciousness of that existence . . .).

Other people are (usually) conscious, so they also create their own existences. That means that, when we come into relationship with another person (or people) both of our consciousnesses become conscious of each other. At that point neither 'my' nor 'your' consciousness is entirely our own because they both become shared.

In other words, when we enter into any relationship, we co-create a shared consciousness, which means we co-create a shared present, which means we begin to co-create each other's futures.

This is a really important point. Being able to co-create someone else's future is a pretty handy trick for health practitioners. So we will explore this possibility from a number of angles in these workbooks.

DIFFERENT PERSPECTIVES OF DIFFERENT RELATIONSHIPS

There is still more.

Because conscious beings live in 'two worlds' (perceptual and conceptual worlds) we can take two different perspectives on any of these relationships. These are relationships where we 'share' consciousness (and so where we can share the 'inside' experience of their existence with them); and those where we don't (and so where we can only describe what we can see from the 'outside').

Therefore, as well as the 'big three' relationships, there are two 'perspectives' on any of these relationships: internal and external.[38]

- The external perspective is often called the 'objective' perspective as it is observation of an 'object' with whom/which we do not have a shared conscious relationship. This is the empirical world of existence, where our existences can be empirically measured, but cannot be experienced or expressed.

- The internal perspective is often called the 'subjective' perspective as it is observation of a 'subject', with whom we do have a shared conscious relationship. This is the qualitative world of experience, where existence cannot be empirically measured but can be experienced and expressed.

A little bit more and we are nearly there.

Because each relationship has both an external and internal perspective that means that each person in a relationship is both subject and object at the same time. So . . .

- Each one of us can be in any one of the big three relationships.
- We can take an internal or external perspective from any of these three positions.
- We can be both subject and object of the relationship at the same time.

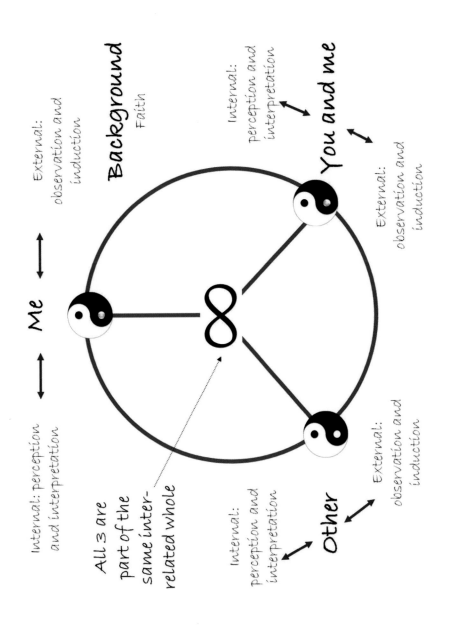

Background
Faith

External:
observation and
induction

Internal:
perception and
interpretation

You and me

External:
observation and
induction

Me

Internal: perception
and interpretation

All 3 are
part of the
same inter-
related whole

Internal:
perception and
interpretation

Other

External:
observation and
induction

This diagram is an attempt to sum up what we have been talking about[39]

> When 'I' experience being Justin Amery, 'I' am an 'I'. When 'I' experience being Justin Amery in relationship with people or things, 'I' and 'I' become 'we'. When 'I' am being observed by 'others' not in conscious relationship with 'me', 'I' am an 'other' to 'them'. When 'other' people view 'us' together, 'they' can only observe 'us' from an external perspective, even though 'we' have an internal perspective, which 'they' do not share.

Finally, of course, we should try not to forget the background, which we tend to find easy to do. None of these relationships or perspectives can ex-ist without something against and from which they can 'stand out'. Therefore the background to our exist-ence is in many ways as important as the entities that stand out against it.

- First, we can't have a picture without a background. By definition, the background to 'everything' is 'nothing'.
- Second, because everything is interconnected and interrelated, there is really only one thing, and that thing is the infinite 'everything' of the universe. Hence the infinity symbol.
- Third, as conscious beings, we can enter one of 'big three' relationships (the I, the we and the other).
- Fourth, each of these relationships can be viewed from two perspectives, objective (non-shared conscious) and subjective (shared conscious). These two perspectives give us two separate disciplines for analysing existence: empiricism (science) and experience (hermeneutics).
- Finally, all of these things are just creations of my consciousness. The universe is an infinitely relational, multidimensional 'foam' of existence, so it is easy to project onto it any patterns we want. The patterns I see are the patterns I create. Therefore, I can't claim that any these pictures, diagrams and words have any inherent existence, because there is only 1 and 0.

WHY IS THIS IMPORTANT TO HEALTH PRACTICE?

By now, you might be excused for asking yourself why we are spending so much time on this strange and abstract concept.

Thinking about our existence and relationality and interconnectedness is actually quite important for practitioners like us. As integrated practitioners, we work and exist within each of these three relationships; we work with both objective and subjective perspectives; and we use both scientific and experiential knowledge and enquiry to analyse things. As we will find out, we are the subject, object and process of health practice at one and the same time.

But we are coming to that soon!

Alas, it is as impossible that my answer to the question 'Who
  are you?'
and your answer to the question 'Who am I?'
should be the same
as that either of them should be exactly and completely true.
But if they are not the same, and neither is quite true,
then my assertion 'I love You'
cannot be quite true either

— W.H. Auden

Questions to chew over

Looking at your health practice, what relationships are you in, and what perspectives do you take? Do you favour some more than others? If so, how might this unbalance you and your practice?

Chapter 6
Truth, language and meaning

Question to chew over
How do you know that what you know and say is true?

Truth, language and meaning are relational entities. Consider this question.

What is the opposite of true?

The answer could be: 'false' or 'unfaithful' or 'unprovable' or 'incredible' or 'insincere' or 'wrong', or several other words. If a word has many opposites, it probably has many meanings.

Or consider the liar paradox, which appears to be both true and false at the same time:

'This sentence is false.'

How can a statement of truth be false?[40] If a concept can be true and false at the same time, then truth seems to be a very slippery concept indeed.

Remarkably it appears that almost any explanation of truth leads to a paradox. Tarski (1956) showed that any sentence has two possible truth values: true and false. Fuzzy logic theories suggest that any sentence may have a continuous range of truth values from certainly false to certainly true.

Any explanation of truth cannot be achieved without some independent analysis of at least one other factor – language.

An adequate explanation of language cannot be achieved without independent analysis of what we mean by language.

And meaning seemingly cannot be explained without some independent analysis of truth.

Oh dear, circularity again . . .

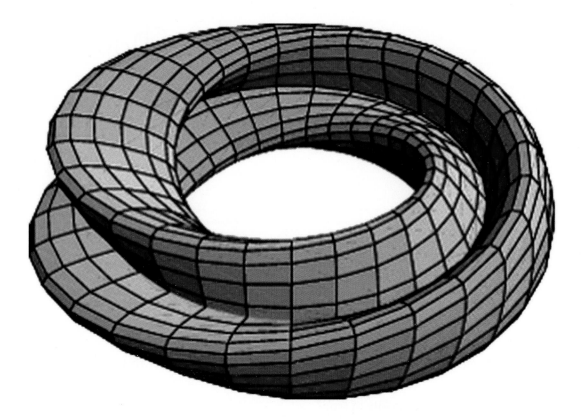

The Klein bottle is a self-referential loop made up of a single closed, non-orientable surface that has no inside or outside.[41] This image is analogous to the relationship between truth, language and meaning. Each one is needed to define the other. We can't get further inside (or outside) than that. We are stuck and disoriented in a self-referential loop.

SOME THEORIES OF TRUTH

It is probably worth looking briefly at some of the many different theories as to what truth is. Some of the major ones are as follows.

- Correspondence theories: truth may be something that corresponds to an exact and actual phenomenological entity, for example a 'hat' or 'cat'.
- Systems theories: truth may be something that can only be described in relation to other statements that appear to be true, such that the whole system of truths create a 'system' within which each truth 'fits'. For example, the classical theory of the universe, or Marx's theory of class conflict.
- Constructivist theories: truth may be something that we construct as a culture or community or family; for example, different cultural 'truths' about what makes someone 'feminine' or 'wealthy'.
- Pragmatic theories: truth may not matter, as long as it leads to an outcome that

is practical and useful, such as money. It is difficult to explain what it is, but we all know how to use it.

- Redundancy theories: truth may mean absolutely nothing, and be an entirely redundant term. For example, we can say, 'It is true that 1+1=2. We can equally just say, 1+1=2. So the words 'it is true that' are entirely redundant. If something is, it is. If it's not, it isn't. We don't need to comment on truth of it.

THE RELATIONSHIP BETWEEN TRUTH, MEANING AND LANGUAGE

All of the theories of truth appear to depend on how we use language. In turn, theories of language depend on the concept of meaning.[42] But then theories of meaning depend on truth, as they are an attempt to convey how things actually (truthfully) are.

Meaning, truth and language are part of the same self-referential loop.

So, are we stuck? Well, yes and no. It appears we can't define truth, meaning and language without creating self-referential loops, but we can find a common link: consciousness. Consciousness is the common factor in the relationship between truth, language and meaning. It is through consciousness that we think, and thinking is how we arrive at concepts such as meaning, truth and language.

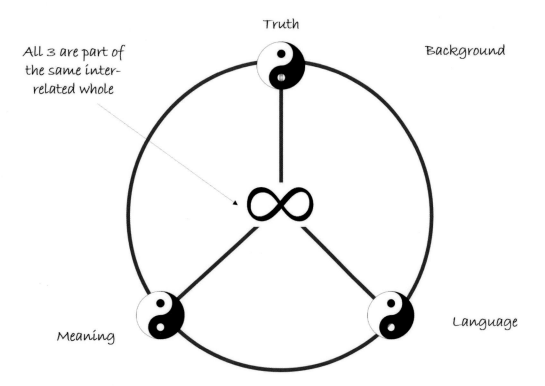

That diagram again, this time looking at the interrelationship between truth, language and meaning

LANGUAGE AND THOUGHT

We have already seen how consciousness is itself a relational entity with no fixed meaning. We therefore may not be surprised to hear that the relationship between language and thought is also unclear and relational.

Like truth, language also appears to be relational, and there are also many different theories as to whether language is created by meaning, whether meaning is created by language, or some combination of both.[43]

In other words, what we 'mean' to 'say' may not be exactly conveyed in the words we choose to convey that meaning, and what is 'heard' may be yet another thing entirely, as the hearer's interpretation of the same words may be different to mine.[44]

This is an example of a common problem, which we will return to again and again in this book.

The problem is that the 'reality' of the universe is not exactly captured by any conscious 'model' we create in our minds to represent the universe to ourselves. Any theories that we generate to describe these models are yet again different from the models. So 'reality', 'models' and 'theories' are increasingly divergent. For these three we could also read 'truth', 'language' and 'meaning'.

THE PROBLEM OF PARADOX

The problem with systems such as 'consciousness', 'truth', 'mathematics', 'language' and 'meaning' is that they are self-referential.

A self-referential system is one which depends on elements within itself to define itself. Within self-referential systems all concepts can fit into a logical system. But none of these elements can prove the rightness of the system itself.

For example, mathematics is a completely logical but self-referential system based upon the principle that x=x. However, self-evidently (and self-referentially) true this may be, we can't prove x=x.

If we try to use systems to prove themselves we end up either in a paradox or in a situation of infinite regress. This is true of the 'truth/meaning/language' discussion, but also in many other areas of human thought.

Paradox

Seeing is blindness

Having is hurting

Hoping is crying

Loving is losing

– JA

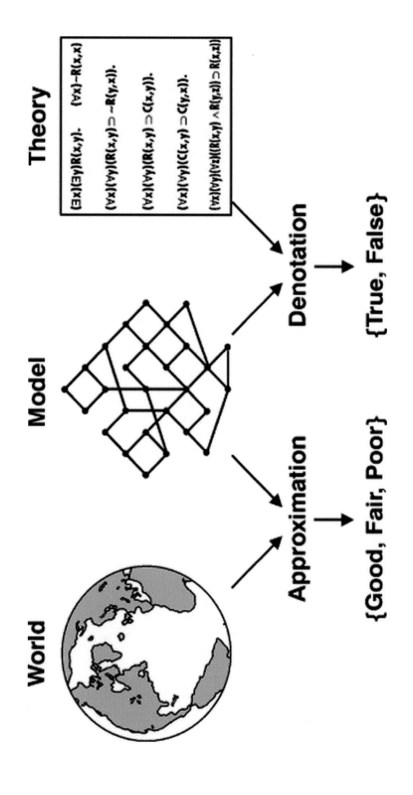

All models are wrong, but some are useful.[45] The increasingly divergent relationship between the actuality, the model and the theory.

IS LOGIC LOGICAL?

When we look into it, it appears that almost any explanation of truth leads to a paradox. Tarski,[46] Gödel, Russell and Moore demonstrated inherent paradox in various different 'languages' we use: mathematics, logic and verbal language.[47]

We tend to think of logic as being 'either/or', something that either 'is' or 'is not'. This 'binary logic' was introduced by Aristotle in about 300 BC, and remained at the heart of Western thinking right up until last century when Bertrand Russell found that, when he tried to reduce mathematics to logic, he kept ending in paradox.

Russell demonstrated this as follows: in a set of sets which aren't members of themselves, that set is a member of itself, which means it can't be a member of itself, which means it could . . .

Interestingly, although this issue has only really come to light in Western thought in the last century or so, in Eastern mystical traditions it has been an item of faith. In the 5th century BC, Lao Tzu wrote:

The words of truth are always paradoxical.

So maybe the issue is the way we think about logic in the first place. As we have just seen, Eastern thought has always been quite happy that things can be both A and not A at the same time.

As a result of Russell's work, in the second half of the 20th century, mathematicians started revisiting the idea that logic has to be binary. This work generated a new form of logic, called 'fuzzy logic', within which there is a range of truth value from certainly false to certainly true.

This again is quite a brain-stretching idea for those of us brought up and educated in the Western tradition, but I gather fuzzy logic works in practice (in intelligent machines) so I suppose, as practitioners, we have to accept that.

IS DISCUSSION POINTLESS?

It appears that any explanation of truth cannot be achieved without some independent analysis of at least one other factor – language. It also appears that any explanation of language also cannot be achieved without independent analysis of other facts, such as meaning. And meaning seemingly cannot be explained without some independent analysis of truth.

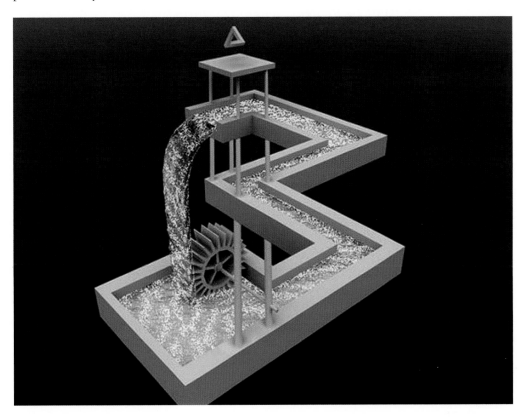

Impossible waterfalls – like this are visual forms of paradox because we can only refer from one part of the painting to another to try to find our perspective. The whole picture is self-referential, so paradox emerges.

It is very difficult even to think about the possible truth of paradox, perhaps because we think using internal language and concepts of meaning. Intuitively, we feel we have an understanding of logic, and that we know the difference between truths and non-truths. It just seems very difficult to prove it, probably because of the inherently self-referential nature of our language, our logic and our thought.

If we can't be sure of anything we say or think, is all discussion pointless?

Fortunately, Douglas Hofstadter thinks not. He suggested that we need some self-referential rules to allow systems of thought to acquire meaning, and enable us to achieve ever greater layers of complexity and development within the same basic physiological systems.[48] Each self-referential loop creates a whole new level of self-referential loops of increasing complexity and abstraction. It may in fact be this very property — the increasing levels of complexity and abstraction – which enables our consciousness to build on the basic foundations of forces, energy and matter to create something as abstract, infinite and complex as consciousness itself.

If so, self-referential paradox isn't a strange or annoying oddity of existence; it is at the very heart of who we are. Without it, we couldn't be conscious.

> *We must not cease from exploration*
> *And the end of all our exploring*
> *Will be to arrive where we started*
> *And know the place for the first time.*
>
> T.S. Eliot (from 'Little Gidding')

A FAIRY TALE TO HELP US FIND TRUTH

If by now you are feeling we are heading off into la-la land, perhaps a fairy tale might help to ground us in reality.

Let's look again at the fundamental relationships ('me', 'we' and 'other') and perspectives ('internal' and 'external') of existence.

If we take an 'exterior' (objective) perspective of the world of 'other' things, we have a reasonable chance of saying some things that are empirically verifiable and so 'correspond' to a particular phenomenon or systems of phenomena. So exterior views may allow 'correspondence' and 'systems' versions of truth and meaning.

Alice laughed. 'There's no use trying,' she said: 'one *can't* believe impossible things.'

'I daresay you haven't had much practice,' said the Queen. 'When I was your age, I always did it for half-an-hour a day. Why, sometimes I've believed as many as six impossible things before breakfast.'

On the other hand, if we take an 'interior' (subjective) view of the world of 'me' or 'we', there is nothing exterior to view, and so there is nothing that can 'correspond' to any truth or meaning. However, there is an awful lot that is within our consciousness, which we can explain or interpret, and so truth becomes constructed, either by 'me' as an individual or by 'us' as a culture. Truth is what we say it is, and cultural truths are the truths of those with power.

'When I use a word,' Humpty Dumpty said in rather a scornful tone, 'it means just what I choose it to mean – neither more nor less.'

'The question is,' said Alice, 'whether you can make words mean so many different things.'

'The question is,' said Humpty Dumpty, 'which is to be master – that's all.'

Or again, if we decide we are being far too analytical (after all, these workbooks are fundamentally about health 'practice' not health 'theory') we can decide to take the view that truth is whatever makes sense and 'works' in the day-to-day world we live in. So if a drug 'works' it is 'effective' and if it does not 'work' it is 'ineffective' and we don't have to say any more about what we mean by 'works' or 'effective'.

> 'Would you tell me, please, which way I ought to go from here?' said Alice.
> 'That depends a good deal on where you want to get to,' said the Cat.
> 'I don't much care where–' said Alice.
> 'Then it doesn't matter which way you go,' said the Cat.

Or again, if we decide that we should only say what we mean, and mean what we say, we can decide to drop the terms 'truth' and 'meaning' as they have no more existence than fairies. If snow is white, we don't need to say it is true that snow is white.

> The Hatter opened his eyes very wide on hearing this; but all he said was, 'Why is a raven like a writing-desk?'
> 'Come, we shall have some fun now!' thought Alice. 'I'm glad they've begun asking riddles. — I believe I can guess that,' she added aloud.
> 'Do you mean that you think you can find out the answer to it?' said the March Hare.
> 'Exactly so,' said Alice.
> 'Then you should say exactly what you mean,' the March Hare went on.
> 'I do,' Alice hastily replied; 'at least – at least I mean what I say – that's the same thing, you know.'
> 'Not the same thing a bit!' said the Hatter. 'You might just as well say that "I see what I eat" is the same thing as "I eat what I see"!'

Or, finally, if we decide to look out at the stars, or in at the quanta, where everything is related at the same time as random, where everything is one and one comes from nothing, we can accept that all expressed truth is paradox.

> 'But I don't want to go among mad people,' Alice remarked.
> 'Oh, you can't help that,' said the Cat: 'we're all mad here. I'm mad. You're mad.'
> 'How do you know I'm mad?' said Alice.
> 'You must be,' said the Cat, 'or you wouldn't have come here.'

WHY IS THIS IMPORTANT TO HEALTH PRACTICE?

If you are feeling increasingly unsettled as this chapter has gone on, you are not alone. Discovering the fundamental paradox at the heart of our truth claims is quite hard to swallow.

However, we might also feel that we have a duty to ourselves and our patients to give this serious thought. As practitioners patients come to us to seek for truth about their condition, as well as for help with managing it. Health practice is riddled with different groups of practitioners making relative truth claims about the benefits of their perspectives and practice.

If we are not aware of the relativity and paradox behind the truths we hold to be true, how can we help our patients find truths about their health that are effective and make sense for them?

As we shall see later, truth claims may also be seen as power claims. Exercising truth claims may therefore be a way that we exercise power, and power is something that we hope to use skilfully and compassionately in our practice of health caring.

seeker of truth

follow no path
all paths lead where

truth is here

e. e. cummings[49]

Questions to chew over

What truths and meanings sit at the heart of your health beliefs and your health practice?

How do you feel about the probability that these truths and meanings may be paradoxical at heart?

Reflecting on this, do you feel the need to revisit anything about your practice?

Chapter 7
Knowledge and intelligence

Questions to chew over

Is there anything that I do not know but which is true?

Is there anything that I know but which is not true?

Is there anything that I believe but I do not know?

Is there anything that I know but that I do not believe?

Is there anything that I believe but that is not true?

Is there anything that is true, but that I do not believe?

As health practitioners we put into 'practice' our 'knowledge' about health.

How we assimilate, process and apply that knowledge is partly affected by our intelligence. Therefore an understanding of both knowledge and intelligence is important to our understanding of what it means to be an integrated practitioner.

WHAT IS KNOWLEDGE?

What does it mean to say we 'know' something?

Does it means that there are 'theoretical facts' that we know, or that we know 'how' to do something, or that we have a deep 'conviction' about something, or that we 'ought' to act in a particular way?

For practitioners like us, knowledge can mean all of these things, as well as the intelligence to apply this knowledge in an effective way. We base our practice on beliefs and convictions about what health practice ought to be; we take many years accumulating and understanding theoretical knowledge; and many more years (if not a lifetime) learning how to apply that knowledge in practice.

It may be quite unsettling then to find that our knowledge is far from firmly founded, our intelligence may be less secure than we thought, and that our application of our knowledge is limited by the kind of situations in which we try to apply it.

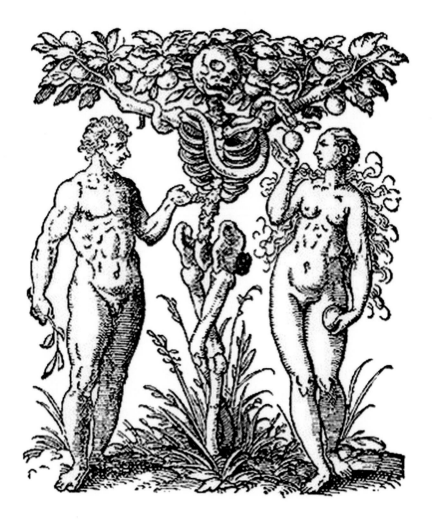

The Tree of Knowledge[50] – it is interesting to speculate on what 'knowledge' could have separated humankind both from its gods and from other forms of life.

WHAT IS INTELLIGENCE?

Intelligence seems to have something to do with the ability to acquire process and apply our knowledge.

We often think of intelligence as something that can be measured, for example by the IQ test. This suggests that intelligence might be a concrete entity which is empirically observable. However, while researchers have demonstrated some validity in IQ testing, they have also shown that IQ is not concrete, and can vary according to time, genetic, environmental and personal factors.[51]

Furthermore, it is not clear how many 'intelligences' we have. Different writers have suggested that we have many[52] (for example, logical, linguistic, spatial, musical, bodily, interpersonal, intrapersonal, creative, spiritual, moral and sexual), and that we can 'develop' along each of these lines of intelligence at different rates and reach different levels.

WHAT IS THE RELATIONSHIP BETWEEN TRUTH, BELIEF AND KNOWLEDGE?

We usually believe that what we know is true. As we have seen, however, each of these three entities (belief, knowledge and truth) is highly relational and slippery, so it is difficult (even impossible) to be sure of our beliefs. What we may be able to say with reasonable confidence is that there is a continuous relational dance between what we know, what we believe and what is true. Each one depends on the other.

Let's have a look at this in a little more detail.

To confirm whether what we believe we know is true we have to 'justify' those beliefs and knowledge in order to obtain 'independent verification'. Sadly, it appears that even this is beset by difficulty.[53]

Let's go back and reflect again on the 'questions to chew over' from the beginning of this chapter (*if you get stuck, you can find some of my own answers in the endnotes*).[54]

- Is there anything that I do not know but which is true?
- Is there anything that I know but which is not true?
- Is there anything that I believe but I do not know?
- Is there anything that I know but that I do not believe?
- Is there anything that I believe but that is not true?
- Is there anything that is true, but that I do not believe?

Without any clear starting point, we have no justifications upon which to base our justifications. We are left with an 'infinite regress' of justification upon justification.

For that reason, many philosophers believe that we cannot be absolutely sure about, or 'know', anything at all. Everything is based upon something else, and there is no beginning and no end to the infinite relationality.

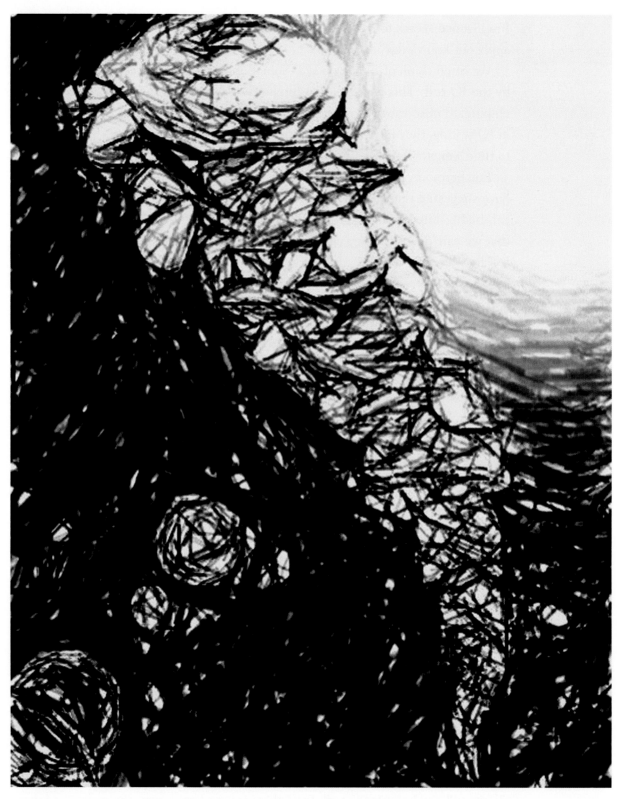

There is an apocryphal story about a guru who was asked by a king what the earth rests upon. The guru explained that the earth is supported on the back of a tiger. When asked what supports the tiger, he explained that it stands upon an elephant. When asked what supports the elephant, he explained that it stands upon a turtle. When asked what supports the giant turtle, he answered: 'Ah, after that, it is turtles all the way down.'

WHAT ARE THE FOUNDATIONS OF KNOWLEDGE?

Perhaps not surprisingly, theories of knowledge echo theories of truth.

As we have seen, we can't truly know what knowledge 'is', so let's avoid that. Instead let's discuss what knowledge can be seen 'as', from different perspectives.

- Knowledge as something that is directly and personally experienced through consciousness: this is called 'experiential' (or 'hermeneutic') knowledge; and was probably the first form of knowledge of human consciousness. It is the foundation of the arts, mystical and contemplative experience, as well as psychoanalytical (particularly Jungian) psychological approaches. It is a fundamental form of knowledge; achieved through awareness and reflection on one's own existence. It is therefore the 'self' in communication with the 'self' (or indeed the universe in communication with the universe). However, it is entirely unprovable, as it is entirely reflexive. It is also very difficult for others to 'know' what I 'know', except through the interpersonal communication, which is always limited at communicating meaning.

- Knowledge as something we observe and learn through experimentation:[55] this is called associative or 'inductive' knowledge. It is the foundation of science and was the foundation also for the 'modern age'. From our observations of the universe we suggest 'hypotheses' which we then try to prove or disprove using fair testing and logical reasoning. We can trust our senses to a large extent, and the scientific disciplines have given us incredible insights into our universe; as well as the technology to dramatically improve (and destroy) our existences. However, as we saw in Chapter 4, our senses can also give us a 'false' picture of the 'reality' of the universe (and our senses may even influence what is happening at a quantum level, just through the very act of sensing). Furthermore, it fails to take into account the subjectivity of all 'observation'.

- Knowledge as something that is a construction of the cultures that we live in: this is called 'constructed' knowledge. It is the foundation of some social sciences and humanities (although these also use empirical approaches to knowledge too). It is also the foundation of the 'post-modern age'. It highlights the subjective and inter-subjective nature of knowledge, as well as making clear that knowledge and power are unavoidably intertwined (most knowledge claims are also power claims). However, without some grounding in 'objectivity', pure constructivism can become absolute relativism, which suggests that all truth is relative and therefore the value we ascribe to different truths is simply a subjective reflection of self-interest.

- Knowledge as something we 'ought' to do: this is called 'prescriptive' or 'moral' knowledge. It is the foundation of ethics and the behavioural aspects of humanism and religion. It thinks forward rather than backward, attempting to underpin and direct our action towards 'good' outcomes and away from 'bad' outcomes. However, as it is impossible to be sure what is 'good' and what is 'bad', moral knowledge tends to be subjective and difficult to generalise.

- Knowledge as something we work out in logical steps from first principles: This is called prepositional or 'deductive' knowledge,[56] and has been around since classical times. It is the foundation of mathematics and deductive logic and so, as most knowledge systems use logical deduction at some point, propositional knowledge permeates other forms of knowledge too. However, as Gödel showed, 'first principles' of logical systems are not provable by logical systems, and so all propositional knowledge is ultimately based upon a statement of belief (even if that belief is as simple as 1=1).

If we think about it, our 'knowledge' of health and health practice is an amalgam of all of these. Health is something we experience personally. However, as scientists, we also observe, test and experiment with different forms of assessment and treatment. How we view health is partly constructed by the beliefs systems and traditions of our families, societies and cultures. Whichever perspective we use, our practice builds on what we think or find using logical steps, trying to arrive at rational and consistent practical outcomes. In trying to decide which outcomes are the 'right' outcomes, we use moral judgements about what is 'best'.

KNOWLEDGE AND POWER

Knowledge which does not tell us what we 'ought' to do may appear to be of limited use. Unfortunately, as Hume demonstrated, there is actually no logical link between what 'I know' and what 'you ought' to do.[57]

This brings us to a crucial (but little recognised) feature of knowledge in health practice.

Knowledge is a form of power, and knowledge claims are usually (at least partly), power claims. Each of us is always an agent of some vested interest, even if that vested interest is just ourselves.

Foucault was one of the first writers to demonstrate the close association between knowledge and power; and to emphasise the fundamental subjectivity and inter-subjectivity of all knowledge. Of very important note for health practitioners like us, one of the most systematic abuses of knowledge as power that Foucault looked at was that of health professionals. In the *History of Madness* (Foucault 2006) he demonstrates that approaches to the care of 'madness' are inextricably bound up with control and power of whatever the current, conventional morality of the time and location happens to be.

Knowledge which we use to tell other people what they 'ought' to do is very dangerous knowledge indeed. It is neither benign nor academic. It is a weapon with which to fight for our interests, consciously or subconsciously. Like all weapons, whether we use it effectively or not takes insight, awareness and training.

This is a very important insight for health practitioners, who are often called upon by patients to offer advice on what they 'ought' to do, but who are also usually 'agents'

of other interests (for example, the state, academia, religious groups, biopharmaco-
logical industry, the bourgeoisie and ourselves).

It is quite sobering to think how often we tell patients what we 'ought' to do, without making absolutely clear who else (apart from the patient) stands to gain.

> For example, with my family practitioner hat on I may often encourage people to stop smoking – a classical 'ought' statement. My 'reasoning' usually goes something like this (although hopefully with a little more gentle tact)!
> - You smoke – TRUE – this is an 'is' statement of fact (assuming the patient confesses!)
> - Smoking causes cancer – NOT TRUE. We can only say that empirical evidence strongly suggests that smoking causes cancer.
> - So you ought to stop smoking – NOT TRUE. There is no logical connection between the assertion that smoking appears to cause cancer and that the patient *ought* to stop. My claim that my patient should stop smoking is partly a power claim (I know what is best for you) and is also partly influenced by subjective and self-interested influences (such as my medicalised view of health, the grounding belief that health is worth more than pleasure and the simple fact my pay is at least partly related to my success in stopping people smoking).

HOW DO WE APPLY OUR KNOWLEDGE IN PRACTICE?

We may sometimes fall into thinking that only one form of knowledge is 'right'. This is called a 'mono-logical' approach.

In fact, over the period of human history, several different 'mono-logical' views have come to the top of the 'power tree' (and dropped down it again); for example, deductive knowledge in the classical era, metaphysical knowledge through antiquity to the Renaissance era, empirical inductive knowledge in the modern era, and constructed knowledge in the post-modern era.[58]

We become aware that each form of 'knowledge' has strengths and weaknesses. As health practitioners we may sometimes be tempted into a mono-logical approach: nailing our colours to one particular mast, and choosing a particular approach we think is most effective. For example, sometimes we label ourselves 'Western' or 'traditional' or 'evidence-based', or 'holistic', or 'grounded' practitioners.

An alternative approach is to take a 'multi-logical' view, that each form of knowledge is useful, when applied to the appropriate perspective and relationship. This would be the approach of the 'integrated practitioner', as it accepts the value and limitations of each approach.

Looking back at our three relationships, a method of 'using' knowledge most logically is as follows.
- From the perspective of 'me': experiential knowledge offers our patients (and

ourselves) an opportunity to learn more about our own experiences and existences, and learn to express these existences in ways that are more 'healthy'.

● From the perspective of 'we': constructed knowledge offers our patients (and ourselves) an opportunity to learn more about our existences within a multidimensional, multifaceted and inter-subjective cultural whole, so we can find and construct a more 'healthy' existence.

● From the perspective of 'other': inductive knowledge offers our patients and ourselves perspectives and tools to assess, analyse and alter our existences as physical entities within a physical universe, so that our physical existences are as healthily effective as possible.

As to where we 'ought' to go, that is a question of belief as much as knowledge.

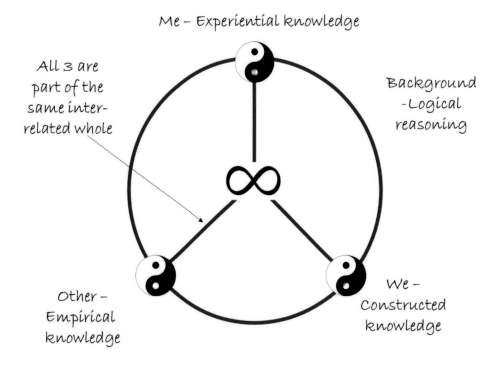

WHY IS THIS IMPORTANT TO HEALTH PRACTICE?

By being aware of the different forms of knowledge, and the appropriate form of enquiry for each different relationship and perspective, we can significantly broaden our skills as practitioners, using empirical, constructed and metaphysical approaches as the situation demands.

In applying these different forms of knowledge, we can become more aware of the ultimate beliefs upon which we are basing our knowledge claims; and then use careful deductive logic to try to apply these knowledge claims as effectively as possible.

In making knowledge claims about what patients (or students, or staff, or colleagues) 'ought' to do, we can also try to become more aware about what power claims we are simultaneously making, so that we can try to balance these claims as far towards the interests of our patients as we possibly can.

Finally, as integrated practitioners, we can be aware of the background perspective of nothingness, which helps us to remember that, we 'see through a glass but darkly'. At the heart of all knowledge systems is self-referential paradox.

> *The only true wisdom is in knowing you know nothing.*
>
> – Socrates

If we wish to be wise practitioners as well as integrated practitioners, we may wish also to become aware of the 'knowledge' that, ultimately, whatever we think we know, we know nothing.

All is Truth

O ME, man of slack faith so long!

Standing aloof—denying portions so long;

Only aware to-day of compact, all-diffused truth;

Discovering to-day there is no lie, or form of lie, and can be
   none, but grows as
inevitably
upon
itself as the truth does upon itself,

Or as any law of the earth, or any natural production of the
   earth does.

(This is curious, and may not be realized immediately—But
   it must be realized;
I feel in myself that I represent falsehoods equally with the
   rest,
And that the universe does.)

Where has fail'd a perfect return, indifferent of lies or the
   truth?

Is it upon the ground, or in water or fire? or in the spirit of
* man? or in the meat and*
blood?

Meditating among liars, and retreating sternly into myself, I
* see that there are really no*
liars or
lies after all,
And that nothing fails its perfect return—And that what are
* called lies are perfect*
returns,
And that each thing exactly represents itself, and what has
* preceded it,*
And that the truth includes all, and is compact, just as
* much as space is compact,*
And that there is no flaw or vacuum in the amount of the
* truth—but that all is truth*
without
exception;
And henceforth I will go celebrate anything I see or am,
And sing and laugh, and deny nothing.

Walt Whitman

Question to chew over

Consider what you know.

How do you express that knowledge in practice?

Chapter 8

Health and health practice

Questions to chew over

What do you believe health is?

How does this belief impact on your health practice?

WHAT IS HEALTH?

Rather worryingly for health practitioners like us, it turns out to be remarkably difficult to say what health actually 'is'. Like other 'truths', it refers to something without any objective existence. We cannot point at something passing our window and say, 'Look, there goes health.'

The World Health Organization defines health as 'a state of complete physical, mental, and social well-being and not merely the absence of disease or infirmity'.

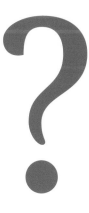

Health

This is probably the most widespread definition of health, and there have been many over the years.[59] However, the definition asks more questions than it answers. What are 'physical and mental', and how are they different? Why is 'social' included but 'spiritual' or 'cultural' not? Who is to say what 'well-being' is, and how will they ground their definition? What are 'disease' and 'infirmity' and how, if at all, are they different? Is health a 'noun' (in some way a state of being), or is it a verb (the continuous and dynamic interplay between different relational entities) or somehow both?

If you are getting a sense of *déjà vu* here, you are not the only one. This is another example of the 'truth-language-meaning' dilemma. We are using definitions to define our definitions, and rapidly going round in circles. Ultimately, 'health' is an infinite concept, and so no more definable than 'truth'.

WHAT CAN HEALTH BE DESCRIBED AS?

Even though we may not be able to say what health 'is', by viewing from different perspectives, we can at least suggest what health may be seen 'as'.

- From a personal perspective: health as a personal sense of existence or being, which is somehow positive (for example, as wholeness, as well-being, as ability, as awareness).
- From a cultural perspective: health as a socially constructed entity that is experienced and managed within and through cultural understandings and traditions (for example, when we agree someone is 'too sick to work', 'disabled', 'mentally unwell', or 'swinging the lead').
- From the perspective of individual 'other': health as an 'objective' dysfunction at one or more of the relational levels of existence (from atomic, through molecular, cellular, organic, physiological, individual, social, environmental or ecological).
- From the perspective of multiple 'others': health as a condition which either enables us to reach (or disables us from reaching) desired goals.
- From a 'background' perspective: health as a manifestation and/or expression of the indefinable nothingness of which we have no knowledge.

We might think about a range of different 'health' conditions, for example HIV/AIDS, obesity, child vaccination, depression and high blood pressure. Each of these 'conditions' can be seen 'as' any of the possible interpretations above. Depending on one's cultural or personal standpoint, one may emphasise one or another of the interpretations, but it is pretty much impossible to find one single viewpoint that completely explains the nature of the full range of these conditions.[60]

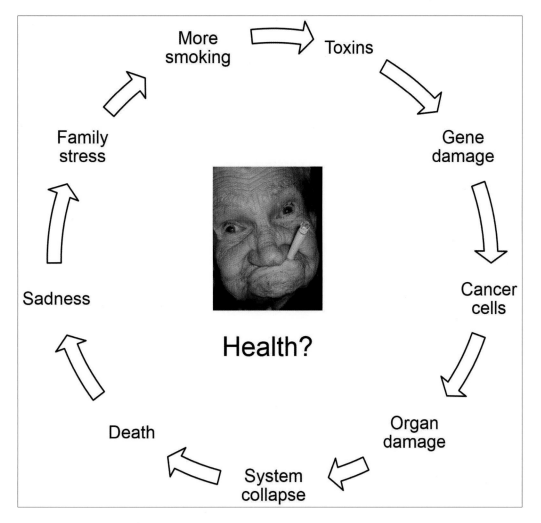

Thinking about the 'smoker' in the diagram above, what 'perspectives' of her health could we take?[61]

WHAT IS HEALTH PRACTICE?

When we set ourselves up and claim to be 'health practitioners', we are making some knowledge and power claims about ourselves. These might include:

- that we have learned a set of 'knowledge' which gives us, in some way, a better understanding of what health is, and what treatment is, than the average person
- that we have learned how to apply or practise that knowledge, in a way that is skilful and effective
- that we can use this knowledge and these skills to somehow determine what patients 'ought' to do
- that we have a value to society that justifies us specialising in, and being paid for, the practice of healthcare.

However, as we saw in the last chapter; if we are completely honest with ourselves and with our patients, we cannot really be sure that our knowledge is founded or sound. We cannot be sure that our treatments will be effective. We cannot justifiably claim that there is a logical link between knowledge of what health 'is' with statements about what patients 'ought' to do. Finally, we cannot easily refute the possibility that our beliefs, knowledge and practice claims are forms of power claims with which we seek to serve the interests not just of the patient, but also of ourselves, and other interest groups that we are more or less aware of.

HOW CAN WE DIFFERENTIATE BETWEEN 'GOOD HEALTH' AND 'BAD HEALTH'?

In the same way that it is hard to define what health is, or to be confident that what we know and how we practise are well-founded, reasonable or in the patient's best interests, it is also very hard to define when health has got 'better'. Without clear definition of what health is or where it is located, we have no objective start point, and so no objective endpoint. Our view can only be biased, partial and subjective.

Furthermore, we cannot turn to the patient and ask him or her, because although they may know how it 'feels' to be them, they may also be unaware of subconscious drives, hidden cultural and social influences, and physical states and relationships that may occur outside their spectrum of ability to sense (for example, at molecular, genetic, cellular or environmental levels). Their opinion too is therefore partial, biased and subjective.

So how on earth do we 'practise' health?

HEALTH AND HEALTH PRACTICE AS CO-CREATIONS

Just to summarise where we have got to so far. We don't know clearly who we are, what consciousness is, what truth is, what knowledge is, or what health is. We cannot be sure that our theoretical knowledge is sound; or that our practice is effective; or that we and our patients are not being influenced by subconscious or supra-conscious influences. Everything appears to be relational, complex and messy.

Does that mean we should throw our hands up and give in? Of course not! We are practitioners, not philosophers. We carry on doing what we are good at. Practising.

Let's take a different perspective, focusing not on what we can't do but on what we can. This is the essence of health practice, and it is what differentiates us from theorists and commentators.

We actually have to do something . . .

We may wish to remember that as conscious beings, we exist within three different relationships (me, we, other) at the same time, and we can be aware from both sensory (exterior) and conceptual (interior) perspectives. These relationships and perspectives interrelate at every moment to create 'events' in space–time of which we are consciously aware. These events are what we call our 'present'.

So, even though our consciousness awareness is partial, and limited, and biased, we cannot deny we have it.

We may also wish to remember that, as relational conscious beings, we **co-create** 'presents' whenever we come into sensory or conceptual contact with other relational conscious beings, such as our patients.

This is something that we are so used to, we forget how momentous, even miraculous, it is. It is also an incredibly powerful tool in the practice of healthcare. This is why.

When we co-create a present with our patients we start to co-create two futures, both the patient's and our own. So our actions 'now' can have profound effects on the 'future' of patient, and also of ourselves.

When we co-create a present with our patients, we co-create a forum in which we can become consciously aware of how it is to be another conscious being.

OK, so this awareness may be partial, limited and biased, but even so, as human beings we are able to do what no other beings (that we are aware of) in the universe can do. We are transcending our own physical boundaries and 'becoming' someone else; just as they are transcending their physical boundaries and 'becoming' us.

Looking at this picture of 'The Doctor' on the following page, we may be struck by how different things appear. The doctor, with no equipment, in a home rather than clinic or hospital, doing nothing except sitting and thinking, in a home with no electricity or modern conveniences.

Or we can be struck by how similar things appear. The doctor is alongside his patient and the family, sharing their difficulties and their suffering, living in a co-created present, considering how to act most skilfully in order to create a new future that will be most healthy for the child, her parents (and himself).

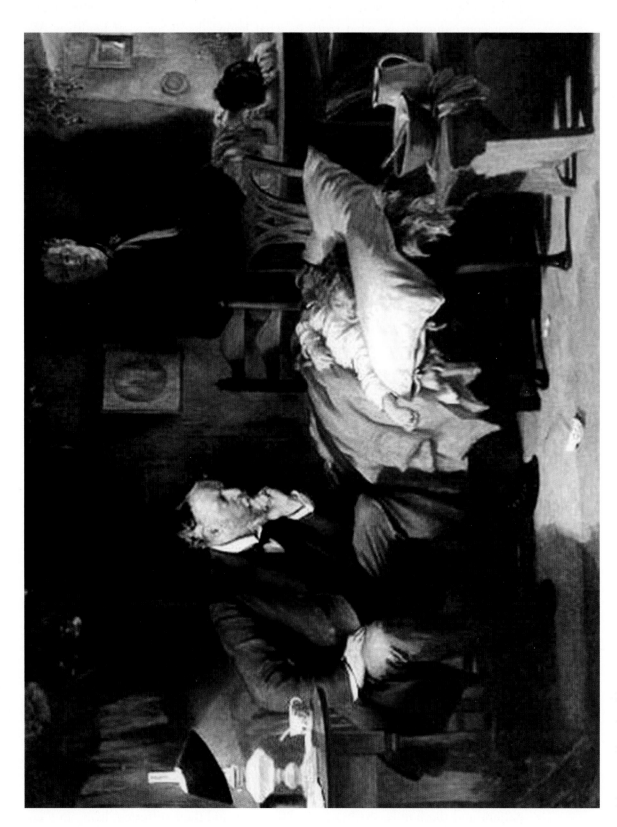

'The Doctor' by Luke Fildes[62]

SKILFUL HEALTH PRACTICE: KNOWING AND BEING

When we become consciously aware of what it is to be another conscious being, we do not have to 'know' what 'health' is or isn't, or what 'treatment' is or isn't, or what 'interests' there may or may not be. Once we are in direct conscious experience of 'being' with our patients, these terms and concepts become redundant, and simply drop away, like silt settling in a clear pool.

This is because we don't need to 'know' these things to be 'true' or 'healthy' in an abstract way. We have the capacity to *directly experience* (albeit in a limited way) how the present 'is'. Once we can experience how the present is, we can begin to suggest, express and test out new presents within our co-creation, until we find one that we both agree with our patient 'is better'. We don't need to refer to any external yardstick to check if this is 'truly' better; because any such yardstick will inevitably be a poor substitute of the direct experience of the co-creation.

That doesn't mean 'anything goes'. There are still things to know, and skills to use, skilfully.

- We recognise that we cannot be sure of our facts, but we can also recognise that, once we accept that our 'first principles' may be statements of belief, we can still approach our co-creation logically and deductively.
- We recognise that we cannot be sure of our senses. But we can also recognise that our senses give us a tremendous amount of information and, if handled empirically, according to careful scientific principles, we can multiply exponentially that base sensory knowledge, and also multiply exponentially our ability to alter 'dysfunctional' physical entities, by creating and using more technologies for 'assessment', 'diagnosis' and 'treatment' of our co-creation.
- We recognise that our experience is personal and subjective. But we can also recognise that, in co-creating, we create a forum within which we can share our subjectivity, our feelings, our stories, our beliefs, our hopes and our fears; thereby co-creating presents which have more meaning, and purpose, and which 'feel better'.
- We recognise that our experience is cultural and constructed. But we can also recognise that this construction is a two-way process. Within our co-creation, we can explore hidden constructions, seek hidden narratives, act out cultural dramas, and create new meanings and new stories that can go back into and help develop the culture from which they come.
- We recognise that 'every-thing' exists against and out of a background of 'no-thing'. But we can also recognise that our co-creation, by remembering its context, its origins, and its destination, can achieve a sense of perspective, of balance and of peace.

This is the transcript of what a patient said to me during the course of writing this book. Consider her choices of imagery, subject, verbs and objects.

What do they tell you about the different interpretations of health this patient might be integrating within her experience of her 'health'.[63]

'Oh doctor, I am feeling terrible. I'm a slave to this pain. I tell you, it's really getting us all down. The specialist says the cancer is invading and destroying my liver. If only I hadn't drunk so heavily! Please God I could stop. The drink's in my family you know. Anyway, I'm hooked on that and there doesn't seem any point in giving it up now.'

What do the different perspectives of health (me, we, other; interior and exterior) suggest as options for co-creating a better 'present'? How should we determine which options we could explore and which ones we should ignore?

HEALTH AND HEALTH PRACTICE AS INTEGRATED HARMONIC BALANCE

When viewed from these perspectives, health practice is simple. We just co-create a new present with our patient, and carry on co-creating until we have achieved something which we can both agree is a 'better' co-creation, or until one of us gives up.

'Better' co-creations can be anything, as the range of relationality is infinite.

However, there are some strong themes that flow through this process of 'better co-creation'.

- It involves balancing and integrating many different entities, relationships, perspectives, understandings and expressions.
- It is difficult to describe what a 'good' balance is, but we all know when we experience balance in our life. We call it 'harmony'.
- Co-creating a harmonically balanced 'present' with our patients will not lead to a 'better' co-created future unless that balance can be integrated into the lives of both patient and ourselves, acting as a stepping stone for whatever presents come next.

Therefore, it seems reasonable to think of health 'as' an experience of integrated, harmonic balance.

And when love speaks, the voice of all the gods makes Heaven drowsy with the harmony.

– Love's Labour's Lost (Shakespeare)

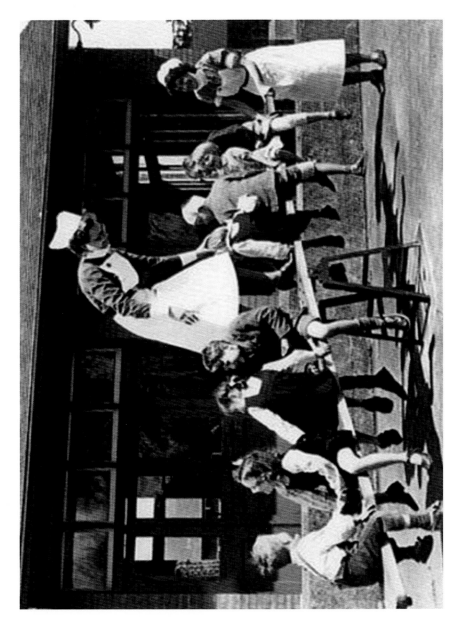

Health as integrated harmonic balance[64]

HEALTH PRACTICE AS A TWO-WAY PROCESS

There is another advantage to thinking of health practice as a co-creation. To co-create healthily, we need the health of two partners to be addressed: the patient and the practitioner. With all of the pressures, targets, budgets, objectives and constraints we face, we can easily lose sight of the importance of ourselves in the practice of healthcare, even though it is obvious that unhealthy practitioners are not likely to be effective practitioners.

Entering into a shared consciousness with people who are (at least in part of their existence) sad, broken or bad can seriously upset our own integrated harmonic balances, and create more negative presents and futures for ourselves.

On the other hand, helping to co-create 'better' presents with our patients can help us discover and create our own 'better' integrated, harmonic balance in the present, and thereby in the future.

If we are more integrated and harmonically balanced as persons, we are likely to be more effective as practitioners.

But what is happiness except the simple harmony between a man and the life he leads?

– Albert Camus

Therefore we have both self-less and self-ish motivations for becoming skilful at co-creating better presents (and futures) for ourselves as well as our patients. This is a continuous opportunity for (and process of) learning and expression that we can use patient by patient, moment by moment. As we seek to create harmony and balance for our patients, and for ourselves, maybe that is how we start to create better health.

Love and Harmony

Love and harmony combine,
And round our souls entwine
While thy branches mix with mine,
And our roots together join.

Joys upon our branches sit,
Chirping loud and singing sweet;
Like gentle streams beneath our feet
Innocence and virtue meet.

Thou the golden fruit dost bear,
I am clad in flowers fair;
Thy sweet boughs perfume the air,
And the turtle buildeth there.

There she sits and feeds her young,
Sweet I hear her mournful song;
And thy lovely leaves among,
There is love, I hear his tongue.

There his charming nest doth lay,
There he sleeps the night away;
There he sports along the day,
And doth among our branches play.

– William Blake

Questions to chew over

In your professional practice, what elements do you try to harmonically rebalance in order to try to create 'better health'?

Why do you focus on rebalancing those particular elements and not others?

Chapter 9
Creativity

Question to chew over

Would you say your practice is in any way creative? If so, try to describe exactly how? If not, try to re-visit your definition of 'creativity' in light of what you have read so far

If health is a creation, that makes health practice a fundamentally creative activity. However, as health practitioners, we don't often think of ourselves as creative. Particularly if we come from a 'Western' biomedical training and tradition, we are

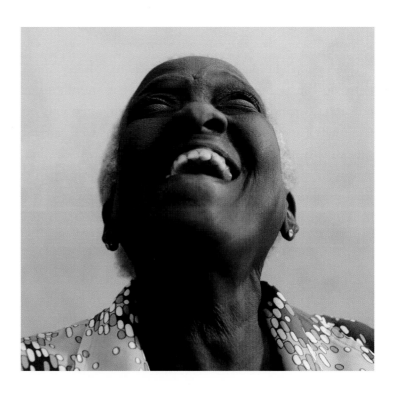

Creating better health: we can't help our patients cheat death, but we can help them to create better quantity and quality of life.[65]

rather more likely to think of ourselves as scientists or technologists, rather than as artists.

But in an integrated relational universe these things are not mutually exclusive. We can be both scientists and artists. Technology can be both our instrument and our palette.

So in this chapter we will spend a little time exploring creativity, scientifically.

HEALTH AS A CREATION

As we have seen through these workbooks, health is a highly complex, rational entity which constantly changes and redefines itself, depending on the person and the context and the moment. So health can be many things, depending on our perspective.

However, we 'know' that our experience of health is experiential and qualitative. In other words, our experience of health is at least partly created within our consciousness by ourselves, and co-created with our patients. So while we can never know exactly what it is, we can help our patients experience more of it. We can help our patients to create better health.

Because health is a highly complex, relational entity, the creation of better health is a very skilled job requiring great craftsmanship and expertise. As we have seen in these workbooks, we have a huge range of tools available to us in creating better health. We have categorised these into 'me', 'we' and 'other' tools, but the categorisation is not so important. What is important to realise is that mastery of all of these tools is no easy task, often taking many years of learning and practice.

We can't each use all of the available tools in our creation of better health, because there are so many. It is not possible to be expert with every tool, and some tools may be unavailable to us because of where or how we practise. Constraint is part of our existence.

We needn't be tyrannised by constraint. There is not necessarily any conflict between constraint and creativity. There are an infinite number of points between one and two; and there are an infinite number of points between one and a million. Creativity is possible in the smallest space as well as the biggest space, and sometimes constraint can be stimulating. And even if we find we are too constrained, that we cannot 'do' anything effective to help this particular patient, we have at least listened and been present. That in itself is a co-creation which is therapeutic.

WE ARE ALL ARTISTS (AND SCIENTISTS)

Over time there have been different views of where creativity comes from. Historically, creativity was seen as something mysterious and divine: a gift from the gods. As we have found out more about psychology and neuroscience, creativity has lost a great deal of its mystery, although by no means all: because it is a product of consciousness. As consciousness by definition is mysterious, creativity will always be at least partly mysterious too.

However, we are beginning to see that creativity is also something that uses and needs conscious, applied and practical effort to be fully expressed; and it is something we all 'do' all of the time, even if we don't think of ourselves as that 'creative'. As Kaufman and Beghetto[66] (2009) have suggested, being creative doesn't mean we have to be Einstein or Beethoven or Picasso. Creativity is a multifaceted thing, available to each of us in one way or another.

So, while we may be technicians or scientists or academics or specialists or generalists or Western or traditional, we can all also create, because creativity is an inherent part of consciousness, and because health is a created, qualitative, subjective experience. To be conscious is to create, and to be conscious in company with other conscious beings is to co-create.

So perhaps the question not 'Is practice art?' but rather 'How expert can our art be?'

HOW DO WE CREATE IN PRACTICE?

To answer this important question, let's start at the end and go backwards. Let's start with our creation: better health.

If better health is our creation, we are the artists and our practice is the canvas. The palette, materials and tools we use to create on our canvas vary, depending on our background, training and job. For example we may create . . .

- by using drugs to create rebalanced biochemical systems
- by using foreign cells to create rebalanced immune systems
- by using encouragement, motivation and behavioural therapy to create a better balanced lifestyle
- by using radiation to create rebalanced cellular biology
- by using drama to create rebalanced relationships
- by using surgical instruments to create rebalanced anatomical structures
- by using narrative to create rebalanced personal stories
- by using technology to create rebalanced biochemical or physiological systems
- by using hypnosis to create rebalanced behaviour and choices
- by using political and public health interventions to create rebalanced populations
- by using physical therapies to create rebalanced musculoskeletal structures
- by simply listening and being present to create rebalanced perspectives.

Our creation 'better health' will vary from time to time, from place to place, from person to person and from discipline to discipline. What I create as a family practitioner or as a children's palliative care doctor will be quite different to the creation of a counsellor or a surgeon or a nurse or a physiotherapist. What we each create will be different from patient to patient, moment to moment. We may be using the same set of tools, but every time we create better health, we create something different, new, that no one else has ever done.

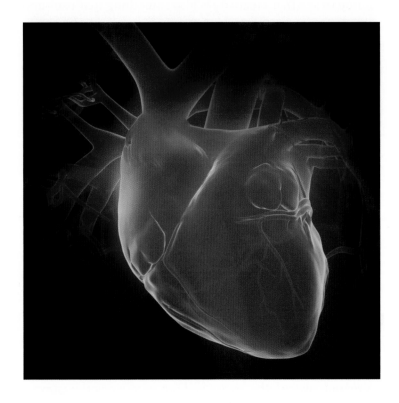

Creating better health: we can use molecular, surgical, radiographic, physical, psychological, social, cultural and environmental techniques to create better cardiac health.[67]

DISSONANCE: THE TRIGGER FOR CREATIVITY

OK, so let's say we agree with the principle that our practice is creative, and that we are artists (as well as scientists). How does creativity 'work', from a scientific point of view?

Well, to answer this question, we will have to enter the realms of neurobiology and psychology. In both of these areas, there is a great deal we don't know, and a great deal of what we think we do know is speculative. However, it is interesting to become aware of some of the current thinking.

Creativity seems to be stimulated and to flourish when we feel a sense of cognitive unease, often known as ***cognitive dissonance***.[68] Dissonance is the intuitive, and often unpleasant, sense that things are not the way we think they should be, and we can't work out why.

Often we experience it as sense of irritation, frustration or agitation.

The theory of cognitive dissonance suggests that it is very uncomfortable for us to hold contradictory ideas or thought patterns. When we feel this discomfort, we feel motivated to do something to stop it. Two opinions, or beliefs, or items of knowledge are dissonant with each other if they do not fit together; that is, if they are inconsistent, or if, considering only the particular two items, one does not follow from the other (Festinger 1957).

Experientially, we have all felt that uncomfortable sense that 'things don't fit'. Presumably (and speculatively) this would have been highly useful in our evolution. If we become subconsciously aware of a shift in the pattern of our environment, and so become edgy and tense, that may have been a very good way for our ancient ancestors to ensure they didn't get caught by the tiger whose stripes in the grass 'didn't quite fit' the normal pattern.

Nevertheless, it is important to note that 'dissonance' is a speculative concept. As dissonance is an experiential form of knowledge, by definition it becomes impossible to prove empirically. By extension, neither can we prove or disprove the influence of dissonance on creativity. However, we can look for associative evidence, and there is some evidence to suggest dissonance increases arousal and activity in certain parts of the brain in association with the creative process.[69]

From a practical perspective, we can say that we live with dissonance all the time. In fact our practice is based upon it. Patients wouldn't come to see us if they felt at ease about their health. They come to us because of dissonance, because of a sense that something isn't right. As such, as health practitioners we are actually very expert at recognising and dealing with it, as long as it is not too intense. We share our patients' dissonance, and hopefully share their desire to stop it.

From one perspective, then, health practice is the attempt to recognise dissonance and use it constructively to create better health.

When faced with dissonance in practice, we have three options.
1   We may try to change the beliefs, opinions or behaviours causing the dissonance.
2   We may try to ignore or deny the dissonance.
3   Or we may try to create or acquire new information, take new perspectives, create new ideas and take new practical actions to create these ideas on practice in order to reduce dissonance.

It is this last option that seems to be the motivation for us to create something new that either 'solves' the dissonance or alternatively enables us to 'see' our existence in a new way that is more consonant with the rest of our existences. Perhaps some people or groups are either more sensitive to dissonance, or more motivated to look for it, and perhaps we label these people 'artists', but creativity seems to be a universal human experience; and dissonance is an experience that is almost universally present in our patients' minds. Otherwise, why would they be coming to consult us?

So recognising, managing and using dissonance effectively is at the very heart of health practice.

MODELS AND THEORIES OF THE CREATIVE PROCESS

Creativity has no more empirical existence than love, truth or beauty, but never-theless it has a powerful subjective and experiential existence. That means that creativity is extremely difficult to pin down, observe, measure and analyse.

We may be able to empirically measure the associations of creativity, for example by looking at which parts of the brain 'light up' on PET scanning during creative action. Or we can observe and analyse different personality types, environments and states of mind to see which favour creativity. Or we can study and analyse the fruit of our creativity, the creation itself.

We can also observe patterns and induce models, trying to create models that best match reality. Over the last century, a number of researchers have extensively analysed what might lie behind 'creativity' and generated a number of models. The first was Wallas (1926). He suggested that during the creative process our minds seem to evolve through a number of stages.[70]

- Preparation: in which we become aware of dissonance, begin to define it and make a decision to do something about it.
- Incubation: in which our subconscious seems to chew away at the problem without our realising that it is doing so. We are not sure why this happens, but perhaps it gives our conscious minds time to 'forget' the previous unhelpful ways of looking at the problem.
- Intimation: which is the 'feeling of knowing' that we are about to come up with a new creation, even though we are not entirely sure what it will look like.
- Illumination: where a creation suddenly appears in our conscious mind as an 'Aha!' moment.
- Verification: where our conscious, rational mind converges on and combs over the idea, looking for inconsistencies and weaknesses, assessing it for applicability and then planning and executing the actual creation.

Since Wallas, a number of different models for creativity have been proposed, all of which involve the result of the interaction, balance and integration of different processes which are triggered in response to cognitive dissonance. These different models have a common theme and premise: that creativity can be explained (or at least partly explained) in material terms, rather than by appeal to mysterious or divine activity. They also seek to understand the apparent paradox of how 'new' ideas can arise out of 'old' neurological processes and memories.

- There may be a kind of Darwinian 'survival of the fittest idea' in which continu-ously, randomly generated ideas compete so that only the fittest are brought to conscious awareness and practical expression (Campbell 1960; Simonton 1988).
- Creative thought may be no different to any other thought, except for the fact we are unaware of it. In this way, it is no different to the mental processes we use when doing other practical things that we do without thinking, like driving, getting dressed, coordinated movement and so on (Perkins, in O'Hara 1999).

- Creativity may be just another skill we can improve by working at it. The harder we practise, the more expert we become, the more creative we can be in our area of expertise, and the more expert our creations become (Weisberg 1993).
- Creativity may be a reaction to practical problems. We create new ideas in response to need or difficulty by analysing the need, surveying all relevant conscious and subconscious information, consciously and subconsciously formulating possible solutions, analysing and choosing the best from these, and then applying that best idea (Rossman 1964).
- Creativity may be generated by the interplay of convergent and divergent thought: divergence suggesting dissonance, convergence analysing the cause of the dissonances, divergence searching for ideas of how to reduce the dissonance, and convergence putting those ideas into practice (Isaksen & Treffinger 1985).
- Creativity may emerge at the boundary of our internal mental representations and external phenomena. Finke, Ward and Smith (1996) described the interplay between a 'generative phase' (in which we construct new internal representations of external phenomena) and an 'exploratory phase' (in which we subconsciously play with these representations to explore possible new ideas).
- Creativity may be the product of actuality and possibility, in the idea that our existence, self-concept and world-view are in a continuous state of self-honing, constantly adapting themselves to new experiences and realities (Gabora 1997).
- Creativity may be borne out of a creative tension or dance between countervailing entities, such as the interplay of implicit and explicit knowledge, convergent and divergent thinking, concepts of 'me' and 'other', and introspective and extrospective perspectives (Hélie & Sun 2010).

CREATIVE THINKING

It seems safe to suggest that creativity involves some forms of thinking, even if we don't know exactly what forms those are.

According to Kahneman (2012) the 'fastest' form of thinking is divergent thinking, sometimes called 'intuition', 'right brain thinking' or 'system one thinking'. It is very quick, creative, subconscious, sensitive to patterns and changes in patterns, and almost effortless. It seems to 'work' by spotting and creating associations and patterns between existing bits of knowledge. It can be misleading, but in the right circumstances can be very effective and efficient. We tend to switch to divergent thinking when we are relaxed, at ease, and have time and space for our minds to wander freely.

The 'safest' form of thinking is convergent thinking, sometimes called 'reasoning', 'system one thinking' or 'left-brain thinking'. It is much slower and harder work to carry out, and requires complete focus to be effective, so we get tired quickly when we do it. It is very sensitive to specific states and builds on known premises to develop logical connections and deductions, infer, hypothesise, model and create new knowledge. We tend to switch to this when we have a task to complete, when we are under pressure or if we feel under threat.

As an example, look at the Müller-Lyer illusion below. Which line do you think is longer?

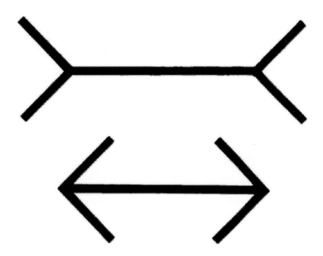

If you have not seen this illusion before, the chances are your intuition will say it is the top one. That's incorrect. It is the bottom one. You can correct your assumption logically, by taking out a ruler and measuring both lines, but that's much harder work.

The elements required for convergence seem to be quite different to those required for divergence. Divergence seems to require us to generate and experience a sense of relaxation and distance, so that our subconscious can flow effortlessly. Convergence is a single-minded, effortful process requiring tenacity, objective and analytical testing, and persistent creative effort to put our idea into reality.

So, again, creativity appears to arise from dynamic tension and the relational interplay between different types of knowledge and different types of thinking. As we become explicitly aware of implicit dissonance we start to diverge from that point, looking for possible new ideas, thoughts or actions that might help us regain consonance. When such ideas occur, we converge on them, checking them for usefulness and effectiveness, and planning how to enact them.

This dance is not so foreign to us as health practitioners. The recent emphasis on empiricism, evidence-based practice, targets and guidelines emphasises the importance of careful analysis, clarity of thought and measurable, effective outcomes in health practice. There is nothing 'wrong' with any of these. We all hope to achieve all of them. However, as practitioners, we are also aware of the importance of being able to imagine what it is like to be the patient, to see the world from his or her perspective, to explore new ways of seeing and managing the problems, and create plans and treatments which will be most effective.

It is not that we can only do either divergent or convergent thinking, it's that we can do both. Each type of thinking can be more or less useful depending on the

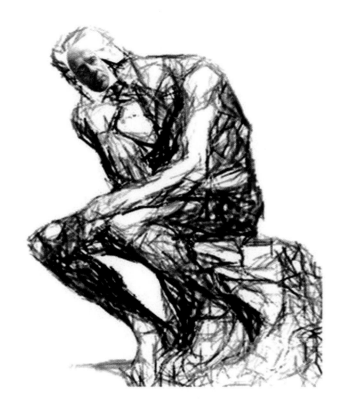

Convergent thinking

situation. Convergent thinking tends to be conscious, logical and effortful. It is the kind of thinking that seeks out and logically analyses possible solutions to problems. Divergent thinking tends to be subconscious, asymmetric and effortless. It is the kind of thinking that generates new ideas and possibilities, often all at once: the 'eureka' moment.[71]

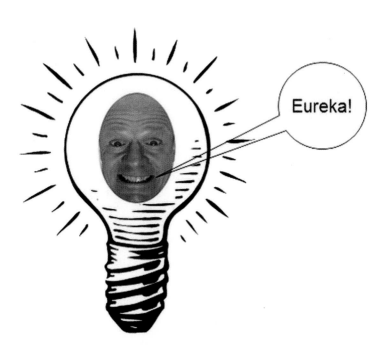

Divergent thinking

Creativity is not just about diverging off so that we can come up with an idea, however intuitively certain we are of its validity. Creativity is also about converging from the many to the singular, about choosing specific ideas and systematically putting them into practice. Once we have had our 'aha' moment, we have a lot of work to do to hone our idea, test it conceptually against our memories and experience, test it logically for coherence, and model it practically, gradually and tenaciously converging on the point where we actually create our creation.

CREATIVE TENSION AND CREATIVE DANCE

The models and theories outlined above have one strikingly common theme: that of creative tension. Creativity seems to emerge out of tension between different values, perspectives, cognitive approaches, forms of thought and preferred styles of practice. It is as if these different entities are balanced and move together in a form of dance.

So how does our brain manage this dance? When confronted with dissonance, the mind seems to comb back subconsciously through previous memories looking for similar patterns and ideas, creating models or prototypes, and testing these models or prototypes against memory to consider how effective they are likely to be.

Different researchers have demonstrated different patterns of neural activation, involving different parts of the brain. It seems that the cerebral cortex may have a role both in storing memories and in generating new ideas, whereas the cerebellum may have a role in coordinating, balancing and fine-tuning prototypes: integrating different inputs from different patterns of activity, from memory and from the senses (Vandervert, Schimpf & Liu 2007).[72] This is not dissimilar to the cerebellum's function in controlling, balancing and fine-tuning thought, movement and other forms of dance.

So who are the partners in this dance?

Perhaps the first is our preferred perspective. As we have seen earlier in the workbooks we can take different perspectives of our existence. For example, we can be optimistic or pessimistic, inward or outward facing, trusting more of our intuition or our logic. If we are too optimistic we may see no need to try to create change, or be too complacent to make change actually happen. If we are too pessimistic we may feel that there is no point in trying. If we tend to be more trusting of our intuition we may find it easy to come up with creative ideas. If we tend to be more trusting of our logic we may be more successful in putting creative ideas into practice.

Another pair of partners in the creative dance may be the different types of knowledge. Explicit knowledge is the knowledge that we know we know: like facts or skills. Implicit knowledge is knowledge we are not aware of, like how we think, or how we speak, or how we move. Creativity seems partly to do with the interplay between these two, a dance between what we are aware of and processes that we are not aware of: our implicit knowledge made explicit, and our explicit knowledge made implicit.

Our memories also have a role in the dance. Creativity seems to involve an interplay between our memories and our presents.[73] Our memories can be explicit (those memories we know that we know), but they can also be implicit. Implicit memories are subconscious and automated, triggering us to act in certain ways without initially being conscious. Implicit memories can also be patterns and associations – the connections that we subconsciously make between different memories, ideas and experiences. As we gain more experience, these implicit associations can grow ever more complex and multidimensional, so that we are able to subconsciously scan incoming perceptual and conceptual data and recognise links, looking always for patterns that fit, and (even more crucially) for patterns that don't fit.

So we come back to the dance between cognitive ease and cognitive dis-ease. As we saw above, when we find patterns that fit, we tend to feel at ease, because there appears to be no threat or challenge that we know we cannot deal with. When we subconsciously pick up patterns that don't 'fit', we tend to feel increasing dis-ease, or dissonance, because we are not sure we are not about to meet a challenge or threat that might overwhelm us. If we are too 'at ease' we may not be alert enough to pick

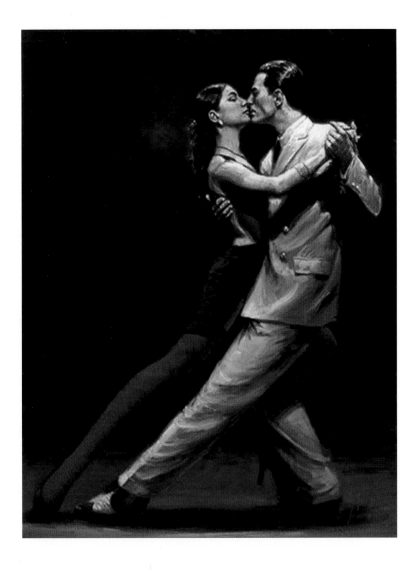

'Tango in Paris II' – by Fabian Perez.[74] Perhaps it is not surprising that dance is a universal form of creativity. It involves integrating and harmonically balancing the tension between different bodies, different drives, different perspectives, different ideas, different memories and different hopes. Anyone can dance, but those people who can dance expertly are also able to create more expertly too.

up on or act upon new ideas. If we have too much dissonance, we may just 'cut out' closing down our creative mind, becoming stressed and eventually burning out, at which point our creativity evaporates.

So creativity seems to be a form of dance arising from the balance and tension between different perspectives, different types of knowledge, different ways of thinking, different types of memories, and different cognitive states of ease. Too much in one direction and we become complacent and stop creating. Too much in the other, and we become overwhelmed and too distracted to create. With the right, integrated balance, we can find the perfect conditions to both come up with an idea and then put that idea into practice.

THE IMPORTANCE OF EXPERTISE

As creative practitioners, in our eternal dance with our patients and colleagues, we don't just want to create, we want to create well, to create expertly.

We may think of creativity in terms of newness, or of having an 'open mind'. If so, it seems we would be right. Being able to see an old problem in new ways is essential for creativity. However, if we think also that means there is no value in expertise, it would seem we would be wrong.

While we can be creative in any sphere, the evidence suggests we tend to be more creative more often and more effectively in areas in which we are already expert.[75]

To understand why, it might help to think about what makes 'experts' expert. Partly it seems to be the generation of knowledge and practical skill. As we do something over and over, we don't just generate knowledge and skills, we also subconsciously notice and memorise recurring patterns, configurations and associations of relevant information. What is more (and we will look at this in more detail in the next chapter) as we become more expert, we also become more expert at being expert, because we also get better at memorising, accessing, retrieving and using that information.[76]

In other words, as we become more expert, we don't just develop expertise in how to do something, we develop expertise in how to use that expertise.

From a conscious perspective, it may feel as if intuitive creations and solutions appear out of the blue. However, as we have seen, creativity is not mysterious. It is the result of the interplay of various neurological processes: our subconscious working its way through our memorised store of previously recognised patterns and associations, looking for a pattern or association that matches the current problem, and suggesting new solutions based on old experiences.

In other words, the more relevant experiences we have, the more patterns and associations we can make, and so the more material for expert creation we have.

This is a really important point for creativity, because it means that, while we may be no more fundamentally creative than novices, as experts we have a far broader and deeper palette of information with which to create; and we are able to use that information to create far more quickly and efficiently than a novice (Ericsson 2006).

Expertise and creativity seem to be relational entities. It is little wonder, then, that our creativity rises in direct proportion to our expertise.

So, while we can be creative on day one of practice, the more expert we are, the more creative we are, and the better our creations will be.

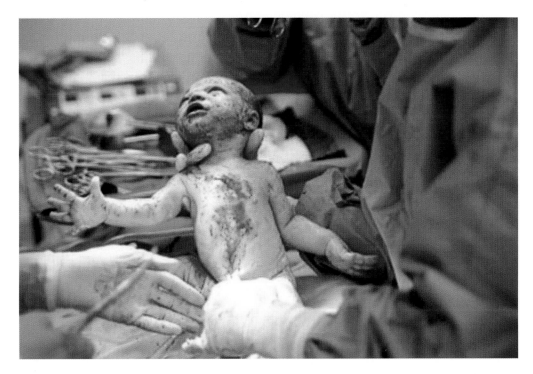

Creating better health: surgery is a highly creative technique, modifying existing or new anatomical structures to create healthier anatomical configurations, and you don't get a much newer or healthier creation than a new life.[77]

CREATING SPACE AND ESCAPING TYRANNY

To dance we need space. Indeed dance is the taking ownership of space in order to create new formations.

Creativity is the same. To create effectively and efficiently, the first thing we need to create is space: space to be mindfully aware of what is going on both inside and outside us; space to enable us to become aware of dissonance, space to allow the tensions and conflicts to play out, space to allow that playing out to trigger new ideas and perspectives, and space to enable us to analyse, choose and plan our new creation.

Unfortunately, as we have seen in these workbooks, space is not something we get much of in practice. On the contrary, we often seem to use up most of our space and time battling the various tyrants that threaten to overwhelm us. There are many of these tyrants and that is why we dedicated two whole workbooks to recognising and becoming familiar with our internal and external tyrants, and converting them from tyrants into tools.

For example, in the world of health practice, we tend to be rather results oriented, looking to converge on diagnoses, tests, treatments and solutions. There is nothing wrong with this. Indeed we would not be very effective if we didn't. As we have seen, convergence is a crucial part of creativity. However, if we are to try to create 'better health' for any particular patient, we may be well advised to spend a little time diverging first, imagining what it is like to be our patient, watching our co-creations, and being alert to novel or creative approaches to their problems.

Being creative in practice by definition involves not avoiding but rather looking for and embracing challenge, dissonance and tension so as to come up with better alternatives. We all have powerful 'internal censors' against this, presumably for good evolutionary reasons. Similarly, because our world-views are also partly culturally constructed and determined, challenging our own world-views presupposes challenging the world-views of our families, patients, professions, organisations and cultures. These are powerful 'external censors' which are also not easy to overcome.

We don't have to look hard to find many of these censors in practice.

- The 'me' self-censors: distorted perspectives, unclear values, hesitant or partial commitment, darkened self-awareness, blocked internal communication, and ineffective action. These can all be made worse by factors such as tiredness, burn-out, low mood, anxiety and sense of overload. These factors make it extremely difficult to relax, to ramp up our alpha waves and to diverge our thinking; and also they reduce our energy and focus when we need to tenaciously converge and create.

- The 'we' censors: inadequate connection and co-creation with patients through poor communication skills. These may be made worse by the sense that we 'ought' to behave, think and act in a certain way, according to the constructions, targets, regulations and cultures of our professions, organisations and traditions.

- The 'other' censors: there are far too many 'other' tyrants to list. Some common ones include poor understanding, time pressures, resource constraints, cultural and organisational prejudice, information overload, attitudes of colleagues and teams, target-driven and safety-first organisational cultures and professional regulations, our working environment, and the 1001 objectives, protocols, policies, targets, and guidelines and regulations that push us to apply singular and simple approaches or solutions to diverse and complex problems and individuals.

It is by no means easy to become mindfully aware of these censors, to find the strength to take them on, and to learn to manage and integrate them into our practice. But we have come this far so we must be tough. We don't give up easily.

Hopefully, by now, we recognise the crucial fact that our most important tool is ourselves. We can create nothing without ourselves. So we are also by now hopefully aware that we need to take care of ourselves. No artist can work without effective tools, and so we cannot create better health without making sure we are able to use ourselves mindfully and effectively. That means we cannot allow our censors to blunt us or our tyrants to overwhelm us.

FINDING CREATIVE STATES OF MIND

If we can create space to create, we can also learn to prime our brains in ways that make creativity more likely to happen. As we have seen, the degree of 'cognitive ease' we feel is highly relevant to creativity.[78] In general, factors that increase our sense of 'cognitive ease' will make us more likely to think divergently, whereas factors that increase our sense of 'cognitive threat' make us more likely to think convergently.

If we drift too far towards divergence, we may drift into unconstructive daydreaming. If we drift too far towards convergence, we will find our over-analysis simply causes over-paralysis.

Convergent thinking requires attention, information, stimulation, concentration and significant effort. Divergent thinking is facilitated by relaxation, quiet, a sense of well-being, a positive mood, and a positive, supportive, encouraging environment.[79]

Knowing this, we can create conditions to make a creative state of mind more likely, fostering divergence or convergence, as the moment and issue dictates. Some of these conditions would include the following.

- The environment: busy, noisy, red and stressful environments will prime us to converge whereas peaceful, quiet, blue and relaxing environments will prime us to diverge.
- Our perspective: to be creative we need to feel hopeful enough to think ideas might succeed, but pessimistic enough to know that they won't succeed without careful analysis, planning, effort and time.
- Familiarity and expertise: the more we feel expert and familiar with the situation, the more easily we will be able to diverge, but the less easily we may see the need for change.
- Substances: stimulants such as coffee, chocolate and amphetamines will make us more effective at converging but less effective at diverging. Relaxants such as alcohol and cannabis will do the opposite.
- Question framing: if questions and issues are framed in a closed way (e.g. where we are using specific algorithms, guidelines or targets) we will be primed to think more convergently than if they are framed openly.
- Mood: if we are feeling a bit high, we will find it easier to diverge than if we are feeling a bit low, when we will be better at converging. If we are too high, or too low, we will do neither well.

It appears that there are many and various factors involved in development of creativity in our practice.[80] But if we can become aware of these promoters and censors, and of the factors that either promote or inhibit a creative state of mind, we have a much better chance of managing them skilfully and using them to our advantage.

BEING MORE CREATIVE IN PRACTICE

Creativity in health practice (indeed in any practice) appears to start when we become more mindfully aware of the various tensions and opposing drives in our practice which may lead to creativity: our perspectives at that moment, the degree of cognitive ease we feel, the interaction of our implicit and explicit knowledge, and the ways we tend to think. Once we become aware of them, we can stop feeling tyrannised by them, and start to welcome them as the foundation and drivers for creativity.

When we have an idea, or an intuition, we are familiar with the sense of a light bulb switching on, or a 'eureka' moment. Sometimes we just suddenly 'know' what is wrong with a patient, or what the right treatment might be, without having any idea of where that knowledge came from.

This suddenness and mystery of creative ideas can lead us to assume that creativity is a rather arbitrary, even magical, thing, which just 'comes upon us'. As practitioners, we want to be practical. Few of us would deny that creative thinking and creative planning can be very useful in health practice. However, if we are led to believe that this creativity is mysterious and unknowable, it ceases to be of any practical use: if we can't learn it, we can't use it, and we can't master it.

However, it seems creativity is something we can learn: we can become more creative as we become more expert. These are all processes that we can become mindful of, learn about and practise doing so that we become more creative in our practice.

Perhaps, most important of all, is the recognition and mindful awareness of cognitive dissonance, because cognitive dissonance is often the first explicit, conscious knowledge that we have that change needs to happen. Dissonance seems to trigger two parallel processes:

- processes in which dissonance prompts us, consciously and subconsciously, to search for the trigger of the dissonance, and to start checking back through our memories for any similar triggers, associations or patterns that might be useful or applicable to the current cause of dissonance
- processes in which the dissonance prompts us, consciously and subconsciously, to use the energy of the dissonance to start to generate new ideas that we have not yet 'tried' but that might be successful.

These two parallel processes seem to dance in continuous, dynamic interplay, with new ideas being checked back for effectiveness against any relevant memories or experiences; and existing memories or experiences acting as a springboard for new ideas.

Practical creativity is neither pure imagination nor pure application. To be creative we need to be able to be imaginative in our thinking, analytical and logical in our planning, and practical and skilful in our application and expression. So creativity is integrated, harmonic balance between different processes.

As practitioners we tend to value our practical skills, which are applied, logical, scientific, technological and concrete. To be creative, however, does not mean we need to get rid of or ignore these skills. It is more that we need also to leave room for divergent thinking, imagination and creative ideation. This creative ideation is what provides materials for practitioners to analyse, mould, apply and express in our practice.

If we want to be more expert in our creativity, perhaps even brilliant, we need to weave together a variety of threads and achieve an integrated balance between many entities: our perspectives, our knowledge, our thinking, our expertise. To get this balance is not easy, because it requires finding a creative tension, and holding it, peacefully and mindfully, while it plays out.

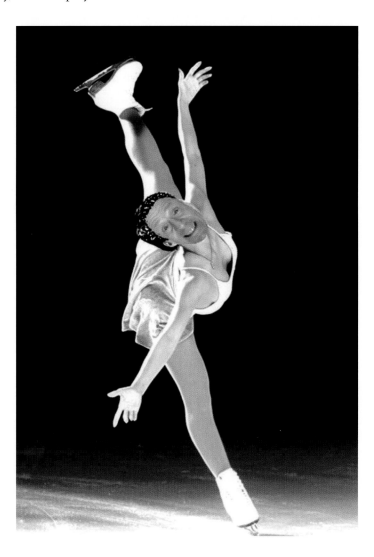

Figure skating, like health practice, developed out of quite strict rules and constraints about what is allowed. From that constraint and discipline skaters have managed to create quite extraordinary and astonishing forms by balancing the diverse drives of the ice, the music, their bodies, their artistic expression, integrating everything into a single creation, moment by moment.

It's not that there are naturally creative people. Creativity is not a gift from the gods. We are all creative because we are all conscious. Yes, we each have natural tendencies and perspectives that might shift the balances and tensions in one direction or another. But we can all recognise these tendencies and these tensions and dance with them to find better balance, because creativity is what comes of that tension, that dance and that balance.

It's not that creativity is easy. It's 99% perspiration. In order to improvise, to head off the page, we need to know what's on the page first. But there is also 1% inspiration. To be inspired we need to create the right environment for creativity to work. Maximum creativity seems to happen when we ramp up our alpha waves: being relaxed, but not daydreaming. What we are aiming for is a state of mindful, relaxed awareness, peaceful, but present.

But it's not all peaceful contemplation either. There has to be a balance. Creating space and time for contemplation seems to enable divergence in our thinking and the creation of new ideas and perspectives. But divergence gets us only halfway to our creation: we are practitioners so we have to create something practical. That means we also need to create time and space for us to converge: analysing, planning, modelling, checking and finally building our new creation.

Wherever creativity comes from, whatever the neurological mechanisms that lie behind it, we cannot escape it, because it is part of who we are. From moment to moment our consciousness takes in an extraordinary amount of information: from the world around us, from the biological processes within us, from our memories, from our knowledge, from our emotions, from our thoughts. Using this information it simultaneously creates the moment and begins to imagine and to model the next moment, always projecting forward and anticipating the future. But the future is an empty page, a blank canvas.

Nothing happens next.

– Zen saying

Nothing happens next. Everything happens now. We can imagine the future and remember the past, but we can only create in the present. Nothing is the inviting emptiness into which we create something. If we want to create effectively, if we want to practise effectively, we need to get out of our own way.

To help us create more expertly we can build our expertise through experience, we can try to achieve the right frame of mind, and we can try to set the right conditions. We can practise, practise and practise. But at the actual moment of creation, we must let go and trust ourselves to create the right thing for that particular moment. And we can trust ourselves as creating is what we do most naturally, and as experts we can create expertly.

However brilliant we may be, few of us can reach the heights of a Van Gogh or Mozart, but we are still all creative, even if we do not think of ourselves that way. What we create, better health, is a brilliant creation which takes great expertise and devotion. To create it, we have to become aware of, balance and integrate many diverse threads. We have to allow ourselves to fall, and to pick ourselves up.

But if we can become mindful of ourselves as creators, mindful of the tools at

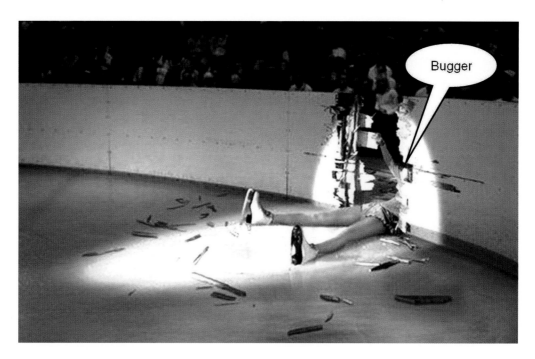

And no one said creating is easy. We fail far more often than we succeed. Failing is how we learn, and learning is an essential part of being happy.

our disposal, and mindful of the importance of keeping these tools sharp, there is nothing to stop us creating brilliantly.

We are all artists too.

Kubla Khan

In Xanadu did Kubla Khan
A stately pleasure-dome decree :
Where Alph, the sacred river, ran
Through caverns measureless to man
Down to a sunless sea.
So twice five miles of fertile ground
With walls and towers were girdled round :
And there were gardens bright with sinuous rills,
Where blossomed many an incense-bearing tree ;
And here were forests ancient as the hills,
Enfolding sunny spots of greenery.

But oh ! that deep romantic chasm which slanted
Down the green hill athwart a cedarn cover !
A savage place ! as holy and enchanted
As e'er beneath a waning moon was haunted
By woman wailing for her demon-lover !
And from this chasm, with ceaseless turmoil seething,
As if this earth in fast thick pants were breathing,
A mighty fountain momently was forced :
Amid whose swift half-intermitted burst
Huge fragments vaulted like rebounding hail,
Or chaffy grain beneath the thresher's flail :
And 'mid these dancing rocks at once and ever
It flung up momently the sacred river.
Five miles meandering with a mazy motion
Through wood and dale the sacred river ran,
Then reached the caverns measureless to man,
And sank in tumult to a lifeless ocean :
And 'mid this tumult Kubla heard from far
Ancestral voices prophesying war !
The shadow of the dome of pleasure
Floated midway on the waves ;

Where was heard the mingled measure
From the fountain and the caves.
It was a miracle of rare device,
A sunny pleasure-dome with caves of ice !

A damsel with a dulcimer
In a vision once I saw :
It was an Abyssinian maid,
And on her dulcimer she played,
Singing of Mount Abora.
Could I revive within me
Her symphony and song,
To such a deep delight 'twould win me,
That with music loud and long,
I would build that dome in air,
That sunny dome ! those caves of ice !
And all who heard should see them there,
And all should cry, Beware ! Beware !
His flashing eyes, his floating hair !
Weave a circle round him thrice,
And close your eyes with holy dread,
For he on honey-dew hath fed,
And drunk the milk of Paradise.

– Samuel Taylor Coleridge

I have included this poem for a number of reasons. First, because creativity is a strong theme of the poem. Second, because Coleridge famously wrote this poem under the influence of opium, a powerful relaxant (and trigger for divergent thinking). Third, because the poem also gives an idea of the upsides and downsides of entirely divergent thinking. The imagery is beautiful and the way the poem meanders, waxes and wanes almost lulls the reader into the same state, but it is very hard to converge on any 'points' or 'meaning' in the poem.

Questions to chew over

What do you create in your practice?

What is preventing you creating even more effectively?

How can you overcome these censors?

Chapter 10

Integrating everything (and nothing)

Questions to chew over

When was the last time you considered nothing?

When was the last time you used nothing in your practice?

We have already touched on nothingness. Nothing is a very difficult thing to consider, because there is nothing to consider. But nothing is what happens next, so we may be sensible to prepare for it.

As it turns out, the ability to embrace nothing seems to be at the heart of expert and integrated practice.

Let's have a look at why . . .

PLATE SPINNING

As we hinted at in the last chapter, the good news is that the essence of being an expert practitioner – an integrated practitioner – seems not just to be about trying to fill ourselves up. It seems also to be about trying to keep ourselves empty.

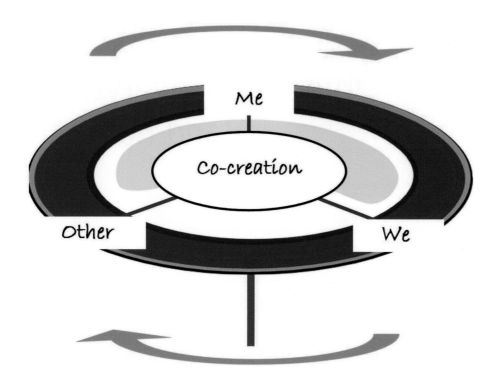

Plate spinning

As integrated practitioners we are constantly in dynamic, complex relationships in a dynamic, complex universe. We are in continuous relationship and communication with ourselves. We are in continuous relationship and communication with other people, for example our patients, but also with our colleagues, bosses, juniors and staff. We are in continuous relationship and communication with a multitude of different entities and issues which may influence our practice (such as money, resources, environment, regulations, laws, ethics and so on). What is more, for each of these relationships we can take different perspectives, internal and external. That is a lot of relationships and perspectives.

A helpful analogy may be to think of health practice as plate spinning. Each of these people, relationships, entities and perspectives is like another plate that needs to be kept balancing and spinning if our 'performance' is to be effective.

No matter how brilliant or expert we are we have no hope of holding all of these entities in our minds. Our memories and brains cannot cope with them all. If we try, we will fail. Similarly, if we try consciously to juggle and spin all of these different relationships and perspectives, we will also fail. There are simply too many to keep in mind and to keep spinning. Finally, if we allow one of the many entities, relationships or perspectives to become too influential (or tyrannical), we will become unbalanced and fail.

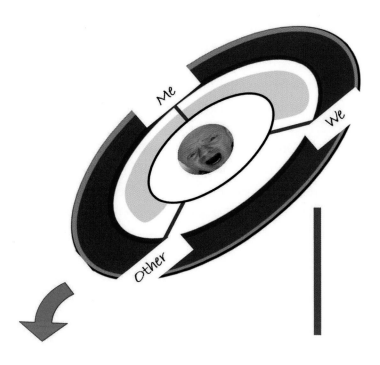

Plate falling

As practitioners, many of us are all too familiar with the sensation of being in a spin, feeling oppressed, struggling to balance and sometimes falling.

Spinning

Switching, moving, running, crying,

Laughing, hurting, smiling, joking.

Hiding, running, feeling, lying,

Turning, spinning,

Who am I?

– JA

Fortunately, we always have open to us another relationship and another perspective: that of nothing.

One theme that we have returned to several times in these workbooks is the much underestimated ability of our subconscious mind to process extremely quickly and effortlessly compared to our conscious mind. As we began to explore in the last chapter, being able to trust ourselves, to let go of what is on our mind, and to free up our subconscious expertise to do what it does best, gives us a much better chance of arriving at a suitable creation, effectively, efficiently and effortlessly.

REFLECTIVE PRACTICE (OR PARALYSIS?)

Interestingly, this creates a paradox, which may be familiar to modern health practitioners, who are often asked to reflect on what they do.

As we briefly touched on in the last chapter, when we become more expert, we also become more expert at using our expertise. All of this is known as meta-expertise, or 'meta-competence'.

In 1983, Donald Schön wrote the *Reflective Practitioner*. For Schön, effective practice is both technical competence and artistic expression. He re-emphasised the importance of learning through reflection, highlighting the fact that, as self-aware beings, we don't just learn by reflecting 'in' our actions (i.e. reacting skilfully to events that we experience during the event itself); we also learn by reflecting 'on' our actions. This is an abstract, 'after the event' reflection that we can use to think forward to similar possible scenarios and adjust how we will behave as and when they arise in the future.

His work was invigorating and thought provoking, challenging previous models that suggested excellence comes from the steady and linear acquisition and application of a pool of expert knowledge.

He was not the first to discuss this reflective and cyclical nature of learning, nor did he suggest that knowledge acquisition was unimportant. But he emphasised that being a practitioner is about being an artist as well being as a technician. He suggested that, as well as studying and accumulating knowledge, we also need to reflect and learn new and creative ways of application of that knowledge by reflecting on our experiences and practice.

His work was very influential, and led to applications in several areas of health practice. These have, in turn, led to many new models and tools for professional practice which have been tremendously effective, for example supervision, audit, significant event analysis, colleague feedback, patient feedback, reflective diaries, and 'PUNS and DENS'.[81]

This flourishing of reflective models and tools has been very helpful. But perhaps the time has now come to ask if they too have become unbalanced, tyrannical even?

Because expertise is also meta-expertise, by asking experts consciously to reduce and analyse the systems, rules and processes they are subconsciously using, perhaps we are also asking them to regress from the automated, effortless, subconscious thinking of experts to the deliberative, effortful and conscious level of beginners.

REVISITING EXPERTISE

Beginners tend to build their expertise in a fairly slow 'clunky' way by learning and then building upon the systems, rules and processes of their profession. As they do so, they become increasingly expert. As we become more expert, knowledge that we initially had to keep in the forefront of our conscious minds (our 'explicit' knowledge) gradually slips from our conscious to our subconscious minds (becoming 'implicit' knowledge). In a parallel way, actions that we initially had to really think about and perform with step-by-step painstaking thought we become able to do without thinking, in a smoother, automated way.

For example, in health practice, we use a number of different processes in our work:

- assessing patients and situations
- deciding what action to take
- taking a course of action (and modifying this course as needed)
- meta-cognitive watching and monitoring of ourselves, others and the situation developing around us as we work.

Eraut (2000) suggests we also use three different modes of cognition, which we pick and choose depending on the urgency, speed and conditions required.

- Instant/Reflex: this is almost subconscious and automated.
- Rapid/Intuitive: which is conscious but only just, as we leap straight from observation to understanding and action without knowing how exactly we got there.
- Deliberative/Analytic: which is when we take in the whole picture and put the pieces together before arriving at a decision and action plan.

These processes and cognitive modes interact as in the table below.

Type of Process	Mode of Cognition		
	Instant/Reflex	Rapid/Intuitive	Deliberative/Analytic
Assessment of the situation	Pattern recognition	Rapid interpretation	Prolonged diagnosis Review with discussion and/or analysis
Decision making	Instant response	Intuitive	Deliberative with some analysis or discussion
Overt actions or action scripts	Routinised action	Routines punctuated by rapid decisions	Planned actions with periodic progress reviews
Meta-cognition	Situational awareness	Implicit monitoring Short, reactive reflections	Conscious monitoring of thought and activity Reflection for learning

As we acquire more experience and practice, tasks that once required deliberative approaches gradually become more 'routinised' and so we become less aware of them. Thus this knowledge becomes 'tacit' rather than 'explicit'. Tacit knowledge is highly efficient as it gets us where we need to go quickly and effectively.

Tacit knowledge is not, however, without problems. Because we are unaware of it operating, we may not recognise when situations and issues move on, so our short cuts become less and less relevant and secure. Therefore, in practice, experts tend to test out their tacit knowledge by generating and testing hypotheses (e.g. diagnoses) or plans (e.g. management plans) against evidence (e.g. from clinical tests or published evidence) or the views of other people (e.g. colleagues or specialists).

Thus practice involves the continuous interplay and dance between tacit and explicit knowledge, much like the creative dance between 'fast' and 'slow' thinking discussed in the previous chapter on creativity.

Expertise is therefore not just about having implicit knowledge and skilled, automated actions; it is also about having the meta-knowledge about how and when to use the different forms of knowledge, different forms of thinking and different forms of action. So the thing which distinguishes 'experts' is not just what they know, but also how they use and apply what they know.

THE DEVELOPMENT OF EXPERTISE

The acquisition of tacit knowledge and expertise develops best in social contexts, where professionals can discuss and test knowledge with each other. It also requires an open and permissive culture of learning, wherein people feel able to share mistakes as well as successes.

Of particular relevance to health practice, time and thinking interact either in a constructive or destructive way. A certain degree of time pressure and resource constraint stimulates and promotes the development of expertise, because it forces us to focus more attentively, process more quickly and adopt more intuitive practices. A virtuous cycle can then be set up, because intuitive thinking and automated acting are faster, so they free up more time for us to meta-process. Meta-processing enables us to take into account such factors as self-awareness, awareness of the context and connectedness of problems, awareness of the various ways we can think about the problems and selection of the most appropriate tools as we practice. Thus our thoughts and actions become more efficient and more effective the more we can meta-process.

However, too much time pressure or resource constraint can have the opposite effect. Once we become too stressed, as we saw in the last chapter, our thinking slows down, we have difficulty accessing implicit knowledge or using intuitive thought, and our actions become more clumsy and deliberative.

Very severe time limitation and resource constraint forces us into almost entirely automated actions and snap decisions with no time for meta-processing at all. Without some meta-processing, we rapidly lose confidence in our abilities, because we have no feedback against which we can check our actions and decisions. In this situation, the effectiveness and efficiency of our work drops off quickly, and we can rapidly enter a vicious cycle: anxiety leading to ineffective thoughts and actions, leading to mistakes, leading to negative feedback, leading to increased anxiety again.

In summary then, Eraut[82] suggests that as practitioners become more expert, the way we practise progresses from conscious and deliberative, through rapid and intuitive and eventually to instant and reflex. In the same way, he suggests that our awareness (or 'meta-cognition' as he calls it) also becomes more expert too, progressing from needing conscious monitoring and deliberative reflection, through implicit monitoring and short, reactive reflection, and eventually to complete, holistic situational awareness.

In other words, as we become more expert, both our expertise, and our awareness of our expertise, become less explicit and more implicit. As they do so, they become more effective and more efficient. It's not that they disappear from sight. We can bring them back to explicit consciousness in a moment. It is rather that they can exist simultaneously at different levels, or 'meta' levels, in continuous, dynamic relationship with each other and with the external world.

We have seen that consciousness is self-referential. We are conscious of being conscious of being conscious and so on. Perhaps it is the same with expertise: we can be expert at being expert at being expert, and so on.

Because our expertise exists and operates, at least in part, at an implicit, subconscious meta-level, we may be wise to consider the possibility that no amount of analysis or modelling will ever adequately capture or reflect the actual expertise itself. As experts we may never be able to access consciously exactly what it is that makes us expert, because at some levels our expertise is a form of implicit knowledge, not fully available to conscious awareness and analysis.[83]

BEGINNER'S MIND: META-COMPETENCE

Let's look again at emptiness.

In these workbooks, particularly in this one, we have painstakingly undermined many of our preconceptions and perspectives. We have systematically taken apart how we see the universe, how we see our own identities, how we view our consciousness, what truth and meaning may and may not be, the subjectivity and uncertainty of knowledge, and the fundamental creativity and co-creativity of existence. We have suggested that the universe is an infinitely great, fundamentally relational and mainly chaotic place, within which our understanding of health is uncertain. From these perspectives, health practice is a massive, random, complex, relational and often seemingly chaotic endeavour, which exists at both conscious and explicit as well as at subconscious and implicit levels.

As experts it is very hard to even remember what the world looked like when we were novices. It involves emptying something that has taken a lot of time and effort to fill – ourselves. But that ability to see the world fresh, as if through new eyes, is at the heart of 'meta-knowledge' and so is true expertise.

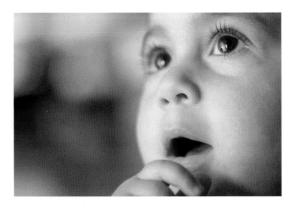

Being so massive and complex, implicit and explicit, no amount of analysis, guidelines, targets, modelling or reflection is likely to capture or contain it. In the face of such complexity and randomness, we are like children. We are meeting things for the first time. We are empty.

Fortunately, experts are not children. Children are what is known as 'pre-competent'. They don't have knowledge and expertise, and they have not yet been taught how to reflect systematically on or to use that expertise. Having expertise is called being 'competent'. But there is another step: meta-competence. Meta-competence involves two things:

- having expert knowledge and skills
- having the expertise in how to use the expertise (in other words, having expertise in being able to access, process and apply knowledge efficiently, effectively and effortlessly).

The importance of 'meta-competence' is emphasised by Epstein in an important but overlooked paper published in the *JAMA* (1999). He builds on Eraut, reinforcing the importance of meta-knowledge (also known as self-awareness or mindfulness) for effective, efficient and expert practice. He suggests that mindfulness is the most important form of professional knowledge, as it 'informs all types of professionally relevant knowledge, including propositional facts, personal experiences, processes, and know-how, each of which may be tacit or explicit'.

To be experts, we need to be able to control and apply both explicit and tacit knowledge. Experts, Epstein says, 'use a variety of means to enhance their ability to engage in moment-to-moment self-monitoring, bring to consciousness their tacit personal knowledge and deeply held values, use peripheral vision and subsidiary awareness to become aware of new information and perspectives, and adopt curiosity in both ordinary and novel situations'.

He contrasts the alternative, more common in junior and training practitioners, who are often so absorbed in the task itself they lose perspective and the ability to cross check and safety net, thereby practising more slowly and less effectively, making more errors in judgement and technique. He suggests that 'although mindfulness cannot be taught explicitly, it can be modelled by mentors and cultivated in learners. As a link between relationship-centred care and evidence-based medicine, mindfulness should be considered a characteristic of good clinical practice'.

So the theory behind 'meta-competence' is that we become more expert in our expertise the more we use it.

- As novices, we have knowledge and expertise, but we use them very deliberately and clumsily.
- As we practice we start to use our expertise more intuitively, becoming aware of answers which are arrived at almost subconsciously, but still wanting to analyse and reflect on what we are doing, not fully trusting ourselves.
- As we become more expert we start to recognise and react to situations almost

automatically. However, it is not that we are actually automated. It is that we have **_included but transcended_** the expertise, to become as aware as a child, all over again.

In the same way, as we become more meta-expert in the application of our expertise, we become more 'meta-aware' of our awareness.

- As novices, we can only take in small chunks of information, and the patterns we recognise are superficial and fragmented.
- As we practise we start taking in greater chunks of information, can process and recollect them more efficiently, and start to notice and use deeper patterns and structures.
- As we become more expert we find we can retain, recollect, retrieve, manipulate and apply much larger and more complex chunks of information; and do so with much less effort, eventually managing them almost subconsciously and automatically.

It is not that we stop reflecting, it is that reflection itself becomes subconscious and effortless.

THE MESSINESS OF LIFE

Earlier in this chapter we suggested that reflective practice can itself become tyrannical, if it leads to 'paralysis by analysis'. We are not suggesting that reflective practice is not valid or worthwhile. It is both valid and worthwhile, if used expertly. But if we get drawn into thinking that's all there is, we could become unstuck.

Reflective practice involves engaging in reflective cycles. Cycles can be useful abstractions. We can imagine and project onto our existence lines, circles, triangles, yin-yang and infinity symbols. These are abstractions which can be very helpful. But they are abstractions, and hence they are simplifications. It is not that there is anything inherently wrong with simplifications or abstractions. Our consciousness is both. But it is also so much more. As we have seen in these books, the universe isn't really like that. It is fundamentally messy and complex – a bit like health practice.

As we have just seen, as we move from novice to expert, we start by looking at surface structures and connections, working through them consciously and systematically. As we learn, it can be very helpful to abstract out, simplify and focus on one part of existence, separated from all the other parts.

If we try too hard to reflect on everything, analyse everything, and model everything, we may paralyse everything. While reflection and analysis have a crucial place in learning and practising, like anything else they too can become tyrannical if we do not use them skilfully. Tyranny unbalances us, and if we are unbalanced, we cannot practise as efficiently or effectively. Once we are expert, trying too hard to consciously reflect may slow us down and make us more clunky and less effective.

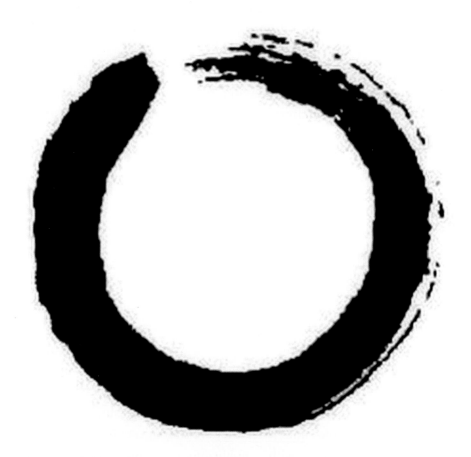

The Zen symbol for nothing – enso – symbolises the moment of nothingness, when our mind is set free from the noise and clutter of daily existence so that we can freely create. Sometimes the circle is complete. But I have chosen the incomplete version, which reminds us that nothing is perfect.

ZOOMING IN AND ZOOMING OUT

This is not the same as saying experts don't reflect, or should not reflect. On the contrary, reflection is essential, because it is reflection that helps recognise patterns and rhythms, and disturbances to patterns and rhythms. But experts can reflect using their subconscious mind as well as their conscious mind.

Indeed in certain situations, subconscious, implicit reflection may well be more effective than conscious, explicit reflection. This may partly be because the subconscious can process patterns more efficiently, effectively and effortlessly, and partly because doing it subconsciously means we are not distracted and so fail to notice important changes or disruptions to patterns and rhythms.

What we consciously 'notice' when there are disruptions to patterns and rhythms is cognitive dissonance. And as we have seen in previous chapters, it is when we notice cognitive dissonance that we can start to create new solutions and better health. This creating involves both divergence (to look for the questions) and convergence (to look for the answers).

In simple terms, if we try to keep all our knowledge and expertise in the forefront of our 'minds', we will be distracted by them, and less able to be aware of, and focus on, what is happening right here, right now. If we can keep our expertise within reach but out of sight, we can really watch the universe with open eyes, confident we have tools to use as and when we need them.

But the crucial thing to understand is that meta-competence is not self-consciously reflective. It involves zooming out not zooming in. It requires us to trust that we have the expertise, and the expertise to use the expertise, but then deliberately and mindfully zooming further out, emptying ourselves, so that we stay aware of our expertise but also so we can see what is happening around us with unblinkered eyes.

We don't stop reflecting. We include it, but we transcend it.

And when we spot dissonance, we re-engage with our expertise, with our convergent and divergent minds, looking to create better health.

BECOMING MINDFULLY AWARE

All thoughts and emotions are things, and mindfulness focuses on the no-thing. It looks for the gap between the images, the silence between the sounds. Once we become aware of that clear emptiness, we can allow it to absorb into our bodies and sink into our hearts, so bringing clarity to our minds.

In the bedlam of health practice, that clarity is a priceless resource. We can use our clarity to become aware of all the sense data we are receiving; to put all our observations into their rightful perspective, and to choose our words and actions wisely.

It is in mindful clarity that we start to flow,[84] completely absorbed and immersed in what we are currently doing. Time and space seem to stand still, we move at maximum efficiency and effectiveness, single-pointedly focused on the moment.

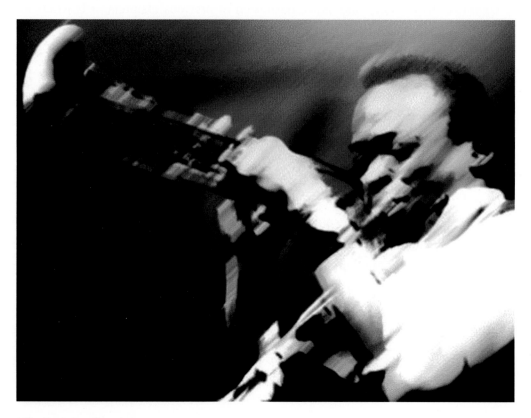

Miles Davis in a flow state

INTEGRATED PRACTICE AS A 'META-LEVEL' OF REFLECTIVE PRACTICE

We are not suggesting that reflective practice is somehow 'wrong'; just as reflective practitioners didn't suggest technical theory-based practice was 'wrong'. The former is a meta-level of the latter. Reflective practice is a meta-level of technical practice.

In the same way we are suggesting that integrated practice is a meta-level of intuitive practice, which is itself a meta-level of reflective practice. Integrated practice is a state of continuous total presence in every moment; and at the same time, a state of being continuously totally aware that we are continuously totally present.

Integrated practice is not about consciously 'finding' the 'problems' and 'solutions' (reflectively or otherwise). It's about becoming aware that the problems and solutions will find us, and that we will find the tools we need to meet them, as long as we concentrate on not stepping on the problems and solutions because we are too busy 'remembering', 'reflecting' or 'acting'.

> When we drive well, we drive subconsciously. By driving subconsciously, we stay alert. By staying alert, we anticipate and avoid problems, and apply the brake more quickly.

Health practice is the same. If we try to do it consciously, it's like trying to drive with the handbrake on. We can do it, but we will be slower, less efficient and harder to control; and our creations will be less expert.

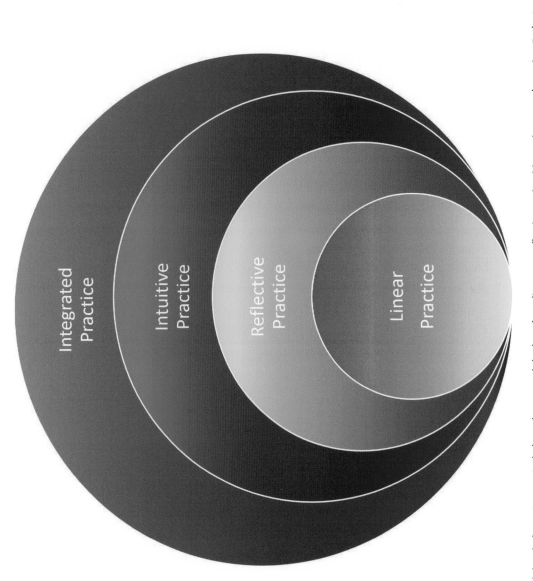

Integrated
Practice

Intuitive
Practice

Reflective
Practice

Linear
Practice

With each level of practice, we include and transcend the last: from linear, to reflective, to intuitive to integrated practice. Each stage is smoother, less effortful and more efficient. At any point you can drop down to lower levels, or reach back to higher levels.

ENDING WITH NOTHING

When we include but transcend our practice, and when we include and transcend our existence, we don't just exist, we also get to experience ourselves existing. We become aware of ourselves, of our patients and of the universe. We get to experience the universe expressing itself through us. We become transformed as the universe shapes itself through us. The universe creates as it expresses, and expresses as it creates. As an integrated part of the universe, the same applies: we create as we express, and as we express ourselves we create ourselves.

The essential point is that everything that we create, that is created, arises out of nothing. So before we launch off onto our respective journeys, it may be wise to pause, to get perspective, and to touch the void.

In this book, when we dug down to find what it is at the heart of our own identity, we never got to anything. We are holons within a holarchical, infinitely complex and fundamentally relational universe, which starts with nothing and ends with everything.

Yet somehow despite that infinite complexity and relationality (and despite our unfeasibly low entropy) we exist as simple, single individuals. We stand out. And we don't just exist. We become ever more complex, creating layer upon layer, holon upon holon. At our highest level of complexity, at our lowest level of entropy, we are conscious. We are not just conscious, we are conscious of being conscious, and conscious of being conscious of being conscious.

From this self-reference we have found only infinite regress and self-referential paradox, absurdity even. But within this empty paradox we have found the kernel of something. This something creates itself, and it lies at the nexus of everything: between body and mind, between verbs and nouns, between language and meaning, between thoughts and actions, between me and you, between us and them, between theory and practice. At this nexus, everything is in relationship, everything is moving, everything is dancing.

It is between the cusps of this paradox, on the crux of this nexus, that we exist. Sometimes the apparent absurdity of our lives threatens to overwhelm us. 'What is the point?' we ask.

Sometimes, when we are weary, or burnt out, or overloaded there doesn't appear to be a point.

We'd be right. There isn't a point.

There are many points. Infinite points. Dancing.

We don't always have to converge on points, aiming at them and finding them. Not that it is wrong to converge. We are scientists. By converging on specific points, dissecting and analysing, we have discovered a huge amount about health and health practice.

But these books have also invited us to take a breather, to regain perspective and to rebalance ourselves. They have reminded us that points are also very good places to diverge from. Sometimes health practice is about imagination, exploration and creation. We are artists too. Perhaps we have lost sight of the essential art of health practice?

Whatever we are, ultimately it all amounts to the same thing. Artists or scientists, we are in the business of creating better health. Better health is a fantastic thing to create. Never mind that we don't really know what it is. We are practitioners not theorists. We will know better health when we see it, because we are experts, and our intuition is trustworthy. When we do see it, and when we do create it, we find it certainly amounts to something, and not just anything, but something very worthwhile.

And the reason we know it amounts to something is because we are intimately acquainted with nothing. It is from nothing that we become something, and it is to nothing we will return when we stop being something.

We can choose to be frightened of nothing and turn from it. If we gaze at the stars, and then peer into the gaps between the stars, and then consider for a moment, we are almost seasick with the weirdness of it. We can't even think about what is 'outside' the universe, because all space is within the fabric of the universe. We can't even consider a time 'before' the universe, because all time is within the fabric of the universe. Fearful avoidance is a reasonable response in the face of this profound uncertainty and disorientation.

But there is an alternative to 'emptiness-denial'. We can choose to see 'nothing' as a blessing and decide to embrace it. After all, there's nothing to be frightened of. Our egos may rage against the concept of non-existence, but the paradox is that without non-existence we could not exist. Nothing can ex-ist (stand out) unless there is nothing for everything to stand out against.

So health is something, and something very valuable to boot. It's not that health is tangible. Although we know it is something, the truth is we don't actually know what it is. It is more of an idea. What's more it is an idea that is different in every person. But this idea has tangible consequences, for who we are, for how we feel, for the quality of our lives.

So we practise in a paradox; existing hand in hand with non-existence, chasing an intangible idea within a tangible life, seeking answers where there are only questions, and suggesting what our patients 'ought' to do when we don't even 'know' what we 'mean'.

In such circumstances it is understandable that we health practitioners have followed our empirical training and instincts and tried ever harder to proscribe health, to measure health, to contain health. In the face of uncertainty it is a natural human reaction to grope for certainty. Indeed, the empirical approach has brought us a long way, and taught us a great deal.

But these books have encouraged us to consider the possibility that engaging with health on a purely cognitive level, or with only our convergent minds, will not get us where we want to go. To go further, we may wish to remember that, however secure, individual and concrete our existence or our health seems, that is an illusion, and perhaps even a diagnosable, classifiable delusion (if we cling to it in the face of the evidence to the contrary).

And the evidence to the contrary is pretty compelling. It suggests we are completely relational, infinitely complex entities, in a completely relational, infinitely complex universe. Health is a subset of both. To find health, let alone to practise health, involves existing and integrating at all of these different levels and within all of these different relationships.

That is harder than it sounds, because our conscious convergent minds are not made for that. But it is also easier than it sounds, because our subconscious divergent minds are. It is not that one form of mind is better or worse, it is that we need both, and a great deal more besides. It seems beyond us, until we remember that it is within us, that it is us. We are expressions of the universe. Arguably, we are the peak expression of the universe. We express it, as it expresses us.

And what we express ourselves against, what we create ourselves within, and what we create better health upon is a blank canvas: nothing. It is the nothing that enables us to step back and to see everything, to integrate everything as harmonically as possible, and so create better health.

These things may turn our brains inside out, but they can give us some perspective and, when we turn our thoughts back to the moment, we do find our mind strangely cleared, and our heart strangely peaceful.

And that's when we can really start to flow.

Welcome to integrated practice!

This Life, which seems so fair

This Life, which seems so fair,
Is like a bubble blown up in the air
By sporting children's breath,
Who chase it everywhere
And strive who can most motion it bequeath.
And though it sometimes seem of its own might
Like to an eye of gold to be fixed there,
And firm to hover in that empty height,
That only is because it is so light.
But in that pomp it doth not long appear;
For when 'tis most admired, in a thought,
Because it erst was nought, it turns to nought

— William Drummond

Questions to chew over

How do you use nothing in your practice?

How could you use nothing in order to become more efficient, effective and effortless in your practice?

Notes

1 The clue is in the title. Practitioners tend to be practical. While we might like to know the theory behind what we do, what tends to be more important is that it works. The original 'Integrated Practitioner' is a whole work comprising both theory and practice. This series of workbooks is intended to be more practical, so in workbooks 1–4 the practice will predominate. For those that are interested, the fifth workbook, *Food for Thought*, will discuss more of the theory that lies behind this work, as of course does the original book.

However, for now, please bear with us, as there are 13 key theoretical points that underpin this work and without which it may not make complete sense. They are as follows.

1. The universe, and every-'thing' within it, came into existence from no-'thing', and may presumably go back into nothing, and we can say nothing about the nothing, as there is nothing to say.

2. The universe and everything within it (including ourselves) is entirely and intrinsically relational. Within this relational web, certain states of matter and energy 'exist' (stand out) with varying degrees of complexity (entropy) against that background of nothingness.

3. Complex entities in the universe are holarchical. This means each level of complexity creates a whole which is greater than the sum of the parts. So, for example, clusters of atoms create molecules, clusters of molecules create cells, clusters of cells create organs, clusters of organs create beings, and clusters of beings create cultures and societies and biospheres. Each one of these can be said to exist on its own, as the interplay of smaller parts, and as part of the greater whole.

4. Fascinatingly, and slightly disturbingly, we find that things that may appear to us to be fixed are also relational. These include knowledge, truth, beliefs, meanings and eventually health itself. Not only are they relational, they are also self-referential. For example, truth is a function of meaning, meaning is a function of language, and language is a function of truth. Self-referential systems always end up in paradox. It is therefore impossible to define with certainty what 'health' is.

5. The universe is made up of the interplay between three things: forces, energy and matter. However, our experience of the universe is far, far richer than that. We feel warmth, beauty, taste, colour and texture. We experience anger, hope, fear, courage, joy and love. The reason that the universe appears so much richer to us is because of our consciousness. Consciousness takes in cold sense data derived from the forces, energy and matter of the universe, and uses them to

Notes

create the full richness of our existence. In other words, and in a very real way, our consciousness creates itself, and creates our experience of existence, as we go along.

6. While we think ourselves as having independent, concrete identity, this is actually just a matter of perspective. From a more macroscopic perspective, we are one infinitesimally small part of much larger relational systems: for example, our societies, our cultures, the biosphere, the noosphere, and the cosmos. From a microscopic perspective each one of our molecules and atoms comes from somewhere (or someone) else and goes somewhere (or to someone) else. From a quantum perspective we exist at the level of probability. From a cultural perspective the words, ideas and beliefs we use are mostly given to us by others.

7. When two conscious persons come into relationship with each other, each person's consciousness creates both itself and the other person. In other words, in relating to each other, in a very real way, we co-create each other.

8. Time does not flow. It is simply part of the space–time continuum. Our sense of time flowing derives from two things. First, our memory links together different states of existence in the space–time continuum in a linear way, giving us the idea that past flows into present. Second, our consciousness imagines future states of existence, giving us the idea that present flows into future.

9. This ability of consciousness to create past, present and future; to create itself; and to co-create others clearly has profound implications for what we think of as health, ill-health and health practice.

10. Health does not exist outside consciousness. It is a relational truth created by individuals, cultures and societies that has different meanings when viewed from different perspectives (for example, biomedical, psychological, sociological, or spiritual perspectives).

11. A common theme emerging from these different perspectives appears to be that health is something to do with the attainment and maintenance of a harmonic balance between different relational entities (for example, between molecules, between cells, between organs, between mind and body, between people, or between groups and societies).

12. While we cannot say what health is, we can suggest that health practice can therefore be seen as an attempt to co-create and maintain a harmonic, relational balance, not just for our patients but also for ourselves and our societies.

13. Being an integrated practitioner involves integrating all of the relationships and perspectives of our shared existence, using all of the tools that we have created and evolved through the history of human existence, to co-create 'healthier' states of existence from 'less healthy' states of existence. Health practice is therefore a science and a technology, but it is also fundamentally creative and therefore artistic.

That is enough of the theory. Let's get practical. After all, we are practitioners not theorists.

2 Edward Henry Potthast (1857–1927): 'Along the Mystic River'. Public domain art.
3 'Ars Poetica' by Archibald MacLeish, from *Collected Poems, 1917–1982*, Boston:

Houghton Mifflin; 1985. ISBN: 0395394171. Reprinted with kind permission of the Houghton Mifflin Company.

4 Special relativity is a theory based on the constancy of the speed of light. This means that the speed of light emitted by an object is constant, regardless of the speed that the object is travelling (intuitively it should travel faster in the direction the emitting object is travelling, and slower in the opposite direction). If light travels at the same speed, whatever the coordinates of space or time of the emitting object, then, logically, space and time must be variable. Bizarre though this seems, it has been experimentally proven time 'slows' when an object is travelling rapidly through space compared to an object travelling slowly. (In fact, time doesn't go 'fast' or 'slow'. It is just one of the four coordinates of a travelling body – the other three being the three spatial coordinates). On the other hand, the 'interval' (i.e. relation) between space and time is constant. By the way, I am by no means a scientist, but I love 'popular science'. A very good and accessible text on the universe is *The Elegant Universe* (Greene 2005).

5 View of Deep Space from the Hubble Telescope (not under copyright). This and other fascinating images can be seen at NASA's website at www.nasa.gov/mission_pages/hubble/main/index.html

6 The second law of thermodynamics is that the entropy of a system always increases or remains constant. As entropy is effectively a measure of the state of disorder, ordered states (such as biological systems) will always tend to decay. Human beings are incredibly complex: holons within holons within holons. It therefore takes a lot of effort for us to stay this way, which we do, as long as we are alive. Eventually, however, as we all know, we all return to dust.

7 'Holon' is a term originally coined by Arthur Koestler (Koestler 1967), although I came across it in Ken Wilber's works. I will be referring to Wilber's works quite often in this book. A good starter text for his ideas is *A Brief History of Everything* (Wilber 2007). A holon describes something that is both a part of something, and a whole at the same time (and often also made up of smaller parts). I like the term as it accepts the fundamental findings of science, that we can be reduced to ever more atomistic parts – apparently right down to one-dimensional oscillating strings. On the other hand, it avoids the reductionist fallacy (which is essentially the idea that, because we can be reduced to smaller parts, that we are only those parts). As we 'know' from our own existences and experiences, the whole can be greater than the sum of the parts. We ourselves are holons, but most complex states in the universe share these holarchical attributes.

8 The golden ratio has fascinated scientists, artists and mathematicians since classical times, as it recurs frequently in objects considered to be of beauty and because of its interesting mathematical properties. It is defined as a ratio within which the sum of the quantities to the larger quantity is equal to the ratio of the larger quantity to the smaller one; and it is approximately 1.618. It pops up in classical architecture, nature, painting, music and even financial markets.

9 For further reading about these elements to the universe two very good books are *The Elegant Universe* by Brian Greene (Greene 2005) and *A Brief History of Time: from big bang to black holes* by Stephen Hawking (Hawking 1988).

Philosophically, it is extremely difficult even to discuss time, as our language is caught up in tenses, which presuppose that past and future 'exist' in the same way as the present. Philosophers therefore are in dispute about whether only the present exists (presentists); only the present and past exist (growing universe theorists), or whether there is only subjective difference between past, present and future and therefore all exist in the same way (eternalists). Whichever position you take, some very hard questions have to be answered.

For further reading on the philosophy of time please have a look at a very good article on the International Encyclopaedia of Philosophy site: www.iep.utm.edu/time

10 From Wikipedia article on 'Time'; image is open source, used according to Wikipedia conditions of use.

11 Taken from Wikipedia, where it was posted by K. Aainsqatsi.

12 'An Exchange of Gifts' by Alden Nolan, from *Between Tears & Laughter: Selected Poems* (Bloodaxe Books, 2004). Reprinted with kind permission of Bloodaxe Books.

13 As John Locke suggested in his 'On Identity and Diversity' in *An Essay Concerning Human Understanding* (Locke, Bassett & Holt 1690).

14 David Hume's suggestion (in *A Treatise of Human Nature: being an attempt to introduce the experimental method of reasoning into moral subjects.* 1739–40).

15 This has been the explanation of Eastern philosophy for thousands of years but has more recently also found adherents in the 'West' (e.g. James Giles, *No Self to be Found: the search for personal identity*, University Press of America, 1997). Religions as well as philosophers wrestle with this question. Western religions tend to focus on the possibility of the soul, although that is an oversimplification, as there are many different strands and threads. Eastern religions, particularly Buddhism, focus more on the 'no-self' approach. This is also present in some Western mystical approaches to religion, particularly Quakerism, which denies the possibility of reducing the self to notions or explaining the self by words. It just accepts (and listens to) the ultimate 'silence' of the universe and the self.

A good introductory book on self-identity and mind is by John Searle (Searle 2004). For Quaker and the wonderful 'advices and queries' have a look at *Quaker Faith & Practice*, fourth edition, (Quakers 2009). Finally, for a lovely introduction to Buddhism try *The Art of Happiness* by the Dalai Lama (Dalai Lama & Cutler 1998).

16 The biosphere is the sum total of all biological systems on the planet. The noosphere is the sum total of human thought.

17 The river photo is taken by Ansel Adams: *The Tetons and the Snake River* (1942), Grand Teton National Park, Wyoming. National Archives and Records Administration, Records of the National Park Service. (79-AAG-1). The image is in the public domain.

18 International Classification of Disease (10) classification F22.8: 'Other persistent delusional disorders'. Delusions are irrational beliefs, held with a high level of conviction, which are highly resistant to change even when the delusional person is exposed to forms of proof that contradict the belief.

19 With thanks to my old college philosophy teacher.

20 Trying to capture what consciousness is and how it works is a remarkably elusive endeavour. However, as we are all conscious, and we can describe our consciousness,

we can say what it is to be conscious from a 'subjective' perspective (although we may have to deny subjectivity exists as well – see below).

21 'Midnight Zen', by Amandda Tirey Graham, http://columbusarts.com/artists/83-amandda-tirey-graham. This is an excerpt from Amandda's thesis about her work: 'Midnight Zen' is dark and stacked with layers of simplistic airy forms that grow in intensity from the bottom up. Some of these forms catch light and rise elegantly while others stay static and darkened by the strange density. Midnight Zen is best viewed when letting inspection and analysis give way to simple contemplation in whichever direction the mind allows you to go. Watch the smoke rise and let your imagination go right along with it . . . like a dream, or a nightmare. This painting – I dedicate to my dad, John Mayo Tirey Jr.'

22 Block (1995) suggests different typology of consciousness: called *phenomenal* (basically raw experience, perceptions and feelings which we cannot easily describe or control) and *access* (information in our minds that is accessible to description, reasoning and control). Other philosophers have argued that there are many more than two types.

23 At each level nature seems to build on the previously evolved level, both transcending and including previous levels in a holarchical way. As each level evolves, so life seems to have become more self-aware: initially through simple neurological sense awareness enabling reflex reaction to external food or danger; later more complex awareness related to pain, primitive emotion, ritual and territorial behaviour; later still more complex social and nurturing behaviour; finally advanced thinking, modelling, planning and testing.

24 A flower is not a flower, or red, until we perceive it as such. Until then it is just another holarchical complex of matter, energy, and forces existing at a certain point in the space–time continuum.

25 That is not to say our consciousness creates the entirety of our existence. Among other things, we are influenced and limited by our physical structure, our biological systems, our societal norms, and by our abilities to sense and process. However, we can never experience these entities outside consciousness, as experience is a facet of consciousness, which is self-creating. While we also physically live our existence within the 'physical' universe of forces, energy and matter, our experience of existence is lived out entirely within this self-created consciousness.

26 'Steampunk – Information Overload' by Mike Savad ©2012, www.MikeSavad.com

27 Language problems again! We have to take real care with the words we use as they can be very distorting. We routinely say things like 'external world' to describe what we can physically sense and 'internal world' to describe our world of concepts, ideas, beliefs and emotions. However, we sense the world both inside and outside our physical boundary (our skins) through highly complex homeostatic, immunological and neurological systems, so sensing is not just a facet of the 'external world'. Similarly, our 'internal' conceptual world *is* the external world, or at least all we can know of it. We are not able to intercept information signals along immunological or neurological pathways and analyse them as raw binary data (as we can, for example, in computers). The 'sensing' happens at the same instant as the 'conceptualising', in the same place (the brain) to the same person (me). Therefore, dualisms such as

mind/body, internal/external, subject/object, and perception/conception are probably inherently misrepresentative and misleading.

28 To add to this problem of circular 'self-reference', our language is duplicitous. For a start, we use verbs or nouns, not both at the same time. Nouns have to be subjects or objects, rarely both. Yet consciousness is a 'verb-noun'. It is the action of inter-action and the state of 'interactive-ness'. It is both subject and object of itself.

What is worse, language is another both/and entity. It may be both a construction of our consciousness and also the inherent foundation upon which consciousness is built and from which it derives. There are several theories as to whether we have an innate 'deep language' which all humans share, or whether the language that we have comes to us from our culture and environment, so we learn to 'think' at the same time as we learn to understand and express ourselves to the world about us.

Language seems essential to consciousness. This is not to say we have to be able to speak to be conscious. Small children are (apparently) conscious even if they cannot say so. It is more that language is at the heart of how we think, i.e. we 'think' in some form of language. It is possible that language is entirely learnt, from our families and cultures, so that we learn to think as we learn to speak. This would be analogous to a computer built with no operating system, which 'learns' to create both its operating system and its programmes through experience.

It is also possible that we are born with an innate, 'deep language' (a bit like the operating system language in computers) which all humans share, from which we build both thought and 'local' language. Perhaps the best known theory is that of Noam Chomsky (1993) that some form of deep language (what he described as 'Universal Grammar') which is hard-wired into young human brains.

29 Edelman 1978.

30 For a good, popular science introduction have a look at *Quantum: Einstein, Bohr and the great debate about the nature of reality* by Manjit Kumar (Kumar 2009).

31 Bohm, David (1981): Also have a look at this interesting interview at www.fdavid peat.com/interviews/bohm.htm. Bohm drew an analogy with listening to music to explain how this might work for consciousness. To listen to music we have to listen to notes from the 'now' and also remember notes from the immediate past and hold these together in the brain at the same time. He sees the notes from the immediate past not as memories but rather as active transformations of previous notes. He also proposes that 'now' is not black and white, but can cover a more woolly entity in which now can extend a little into both time and space. Each moment transforms into the next, with content that was 'implicate' in the immediate past being trans-formed into something 'explicate' in the present. Therefore, our sense of being is an almost infinitely complex interplay of different transformations of consciousness.

32 Many interpretations of 'Western' religions (Judaism, Christianity and Islam) are fundamentally dualist in approach (separating the universe and everything in it into two separate substances – body and soul). However, some Western mystical approaches (Quakerism and some schools of Hinduism (for a good introduc-tion have a look at *An Introduction to Hinduism* by Gavin D. Flood, Cambridge University Press, 1996; or go to www.hinduismtoday.com)) retain this sense of 'oneness', and the oneness is then interpreted as personal (i.e. 'God') rather than

emptiness. Hinduism identifies the 'Supreme Being' with everything: in other words he/she is everything, and everything is him/her (pantheism). Western religions tend to hold back from this position (as it makes the problem of suffering difficult to reconcile with a 'benevolent' God), so the furthest they will usually go is a suggestion that God is **in** everything and everything is **in** God (pantheism).

33 This haiku is a lovely illustration of how our consciousness seems to be. It generates images of sensory experience derived from the physical universe (the frog, the pond, the water). It layers onto that sensory imagery meaning and depth (old, leaps). It creates unity out of subject and object (Which is the subject and object? The frog? The pond? The water? All of them? None of them?). It also creates unity out of the nouns and the verbs (Is it a sentence about the action of jumping, or the action of water accepting and expressing, or both, or neither?). By being both nonsense and yet full of sense it knocks our consciousness out of cosy preconceptions and forces us to look afresh at ourselves and the universe.

34 'Internal communication with other people or things' may at first sound a little odd. However, we are often 'relating' to people or things in our minds; for example, when we think about them or if we remember them. Therefore we are continuously setting up internal relationships and dialogues with people or things as and when our consciousness becomes aware of them.

35 The big three can be found in: 'Sir Karl Popper's "three worlds" (subjective, cultural, and objective); Plato's the Good (as the ground of morals, the 'we' of the Lower Left), the True (objective truth or it-propositions, the Right Hand), and the Beautiful (the aesthetic beauty in the I of each beholder, the Upper Left); Habermas' three validity claims (subjective truthfulness of I, cultural justness of we, and objective truth of its). Historically of great importance, these are also the three major domains of Kant's three critiques: science or its (*Critique of Pure Reason*), morals or we (*Critique of Practical Reason*), and art and self-expression of the I (*Critique of Judgment*).'

From Wilber K. 'An integral theory of consciousness', *Journal of Consciousness Studies*. 1997; **4**(1): 71–92.

36 Even if, to take an extreme example, we were dressed up in a spacesuit and shot off into outer space, we would still be relating to something (either by thinking about ourselves or others; or by looking at or being influenced by passing stars and galaxies; or simply by being 'something' against a background of 'nothing').

37 'Dialogical self theory' (Hermans & Gieser 2011) suggests that the self is more akin to a 'society' that an individual. It suggests we are each composites of many different 'positions' generating many different 'narratives' and so generating a multitude of different 'dialogues' within our apparently 'unified' mind. This allows us to set up and test all sorts of positions and suggestions from all sorts of different perspectives. The downsides occur either when it gets too noisy (so we can't choose and hold one set of integrated choices and actions) or when one voice becomes tyrannical and shuts out or distorts others (an example would be a narrative of low self-esteem, which undermines all other more positive narratives). We will discuss this more in the coming chapters.

38 Ken Wilber (Wilber 1997 and 2007) has suggested a useful model that captures these insights, which he calls AQAL: 'All Quadrants All Levels'. He builds on

Koestler's description of 'holons' to suggest what elements may co-relate to generate the holon of human existence. In this section we are just focusing on his 'quadrants', which can be seen in the table below. We will come to levels later.

Upper-Left (UL) 'I' Interior Individual	Upper-Right (UR) 'It' Exterior Individual
Lower-Left (LL) 'We' Interior Collective	Lower-Right (LR) 'Its' Exterior Collective

Wilber not only describes the quadrants and levels, he goes on to suggest that all human activity and endeavour fits into one of these quadrants, and that we can easily become caught only in one quadrant, or stuck with only one perspective. This is potentially important in health practice, where we are called to help the 'whole' person, but within which we are influenced and trained from particular perspectives or approaches, which can lead to us to distortion and so inability to provide 'whole' care.

As you might have noticed, we are not these four quadrants exactly. Instead we have collapsed the 'individual 'it' with the collective 'its' to create a simple 'other', because there is little practical difference for the health practice. However, if we were to be delve into the theories of knowledge a bit more, we should separate individual and collective 'others', as the theories and models of knowledge deal with these things slightly differently. We will, however, start to include the different 'interior' and 'exterior' perspectives later on the book, and there will be times when we separate out individual and collective 'other'.

39 Ken Wilber captures this really helpfully with his table of relationships and perspectives.

	Interior	Exterior
Individual	Standard: Truthfulness (1st person) (sincerity, integrity, trustworthiness)	Standard: Truth (3rd person) (correspondence, representation, propositional)
Collective	Standard: Justness (2nd person) (cultural fit, rightness, mutual understanding)	Standard: Functional fit (3rd person) (systems theory web, structural-functionalism, social systems mesh)

Wilber suggests that different sorts of relationships and perspectives require that we ask different sorts of 'truth' questions (he calls them 'validity claims').

- From interior perspectives of 'me' we should ask, 'Am I telling you the truth or am I lying?'
- From interior perspectives of 'we' we should ask, 'How do my thoughts and beliefs fit within the thoughts and meanings of my family and culture?'
- From exterior perspectives of individual third person 'other' entities we should ask, 'Does the proposition correspond with or fit the facts as we see them?'

- From the exterior perspective of the collective third person we should ask, 'Do all the objective propositions make a functional fit in the overall system?'

The important point is that all four of these are valid truth questions and validity claims, but it makes no sense to ask the wrong questions of the wrong quadrant. There is no 'objective' measurable correlate of my thoughts, and I cannot ask mathematical propositions how they feel.

40 Remarkably, it appears that almost any explanation of truth leads to a paradox. Tarski (1956) showed that any sentence has two possible truth values: true and false. Fuzzy logic theories suggest that any sentence may have a continuous range of truth values from certainly false to certainly true. Any explanation of truth cannot be achieved without some independent analysis of at least one other factor – language. It also appears that any explanation of language also cannot be achieved without independent analysis of other facts, such as meaning. And meaning seemingly cannot be explained without some independent analysis of truth.

41 Originally described by Felix Klein (in Hilbert & Cohn-Vossen 1990). Image is from Mathworld at http://mathworld.wolfram.com/KleinBottle.html with many thanks.

42 Even the term 'meaning' is slippery. The meaning of a word may be seen as one of two possibilities. It could either be the exact 'definition' of a word irrespective of who says or hears it (semantics). Alternatively, it could be seen as the individual understandings of the speaker (associative). A good example of this is Wittgenstein's philosophy, which suggested the idea of 'meaning as use', and described how meaning of particular words is a community or cultural phenomenon.

43 It may be that we need words to think. The Piraha, a tribe in Brazil, whose language has only terms like few and many instead of numerals, are not able to keep track of exact quantities (Everett 2008). Cultures which don't have exact number words are less able to quantify than people from cultures that do. This is the idea between language control in George Orwell's novel *Nineteen Eighty-Four* (Orwell 1949). On the other hand, it may be we need thought before we can speak. How can signs and symbols (which is what words are) mean anything unless they have already been 'primed' with certain meaning prior to use? Some philosophers argue that language and meaning must coexist, as it is impossible to explain one without the other.

44 Any one thing can be described in many ways depending on one's perspective or motivation, because one's choice of words, and the meaning one intends to be conveyed by the words chosen, are at least partly subjective.

   In *Language and Truth*, John F Sowa. www.jfsowa.com/logic/theories.htm

45 This quote from George Box, and the diagram, are taken from a very interesting article by John F. Sowa called 'Representing Knowledge Soup In Language and Logic', which can be found at www.jfsowa.com/talks/souprepr.htm

46 Tarski (1956) suggested that discussions of truth require us to think about different levels of languages, where each level of language (meta-level) can demonstrate truth only of languages at a lower level (the 'object language'). This removes the self-referential problem, but creates a problem of infinite regress.

47 Some well-known paradoxes include:
- Gödel: if a system is also capable of proving certain basic facts about the natural

numbers, then one particular arithmetic truth the system cannot prove is the consistency of the system itself.

- Tarski: there is no L-formula True(x) such that for every L-formula x, True(x) ↔ x is true.
- Moore: concerns the possibility of language making statements that are both true, consistent, non-contradictory but also absurd such as 'It's raining but I don't believe that it is raining'.

48 Hofstadter (1980) suggests self-reference and formal rules allow systems to acquire meaning despite being made of 'meaningless' elements. These systems are crucial to our existence, and work as long as we work within them. Within complex living systems, for example consciousness, he suggests that these self-referential systems, or loops, are crucial. He suggests that we are formed of 'strange loops' which are strange that they include different meta-levels, or levels of abstraction, within them. So that, as we circle round the loop, we attain ever higher levels of structure, abstraction and complexity but, despite the sense of increasing structure and distance and complexity, nevertheless 'one winds up, to one's shock, exactly where one had started out. In short, a strange loop is a paradoxical level-crossing feedback loop.'

Beck and Cowan (2006) refer to a similar form of development, which they describe as a helical spiral, wherein we loop round continuously, each loop returning to the beginning, yet also conferring another level of development and complexity. He calls this 'transcend and include' – i.e. each time we return to the beginning, we include everything we have learned so we see it again, but we see it through new eyes.

49 'Seeker of Truth' by e. e. cummings, from *Complete Poems, 1904–1962* by e. e. cummings, W. W. Norton & Co.; Revised edition (1994). Reprinted with kind permission of the publisher.

50 The Tree of Knowledge within the Garden of Eden is an ancient story found in Islam, Judaism and Christianity; and may well have been around long before those. This print is interesting as it shows the Tree of Knowledge as also a tree of death. It makes me wonder what knowledge might cause our divorce from our 'God' and our fellow life forms, and which would also introduce us to death. One good contender would be knowledge of oneself as a 'self'. Without that knowledge, we are like animals (who do not – we presume – mediate and theorise about their own existence); death is not something we would anticipate or worry about; and we would be totally dependent on our gods because we would have no concept of ourselves as 'agents' able to grasp and mould our own presents and futures. This print is by Jost Amman: 'Adam and Eve with the Tree of Knowledge as Death' (1587), from Jacob Ruegg's *De conceptu et generatione hominis*.

51 James Flynn (Flynn 2009) is a politics professor in New Zealand. He pointed out that IQ continues to rise from generation to generation, that it appears to be 'multidimensional' (rather than just a function of one single factor called 'general intelligence'), that projecting back in time would means that the average score 200 years ago would be so low as to qualify as 'mental retardation' in current normograms. He suggests that intelligence is therefore a multidimensional entity influenced by genetics, environment, culture and communication.

52 Gardner (Howard Gardner, *Frames of Mind: the theory of multiple intelligences*, Basic Books; 2011. ISBN-10: 0465024335. ISBN-13: 978-0465024339) argued that the IQ test measures only logical and linguistic intelligence) whereas intelligences include linguistic, logical-mathematical, spatial, musical, bodily, interpersonal and intrapersonal sorts. The triarchic theory (Sternberg 1985) suggests that intelligence can be viewed from different perspectives: analytical, creative and practical. Ken Wilber (Wilber 2007) goes further and brings together works from a number of scholars in a number of fields to suggest that there are many developmental 'lines'. These would include all the above, but also others such as moral, spiritual and psychosexual. Cognitive development seems crucial as it is hard to develop up other lines without some basic cognitive ability. However, even so, he claims that we can progress up these different lines at different rates to achieve different levels on the various lines. Therefore people could be highly moral, but not so developed in logical or linguistic lines; or conversely, like the Nazi medical researchers, highly developed logically, but very undeveloped morally and spiritually. Although some cognitive development is needed for all lines, other lines may be completely independent.

53 For many thousands of years, philosophers concurred with Plato's description of knowledge as something that must be 'true', 'justified' and 'believed'. However, in the 1960s a philosopher named Gettier (Gettier 1963) provided two examples in which someone had a true and justified belief that their knowledge was correct (through luck), but these beliefs and justifications were wrong. The fundamental problems are that we can never be certain that what is 'in here' in our minds corresponds exactly to what is 'out there' in the universe (and we can't because the representation of the universe in our 'minds' is not as sophisticated as the reality 'out there'); and also that we can never be certain that any evaluation to confirm that the match between what is 'in here' in our minds and what is 'out there' in the universe has been carried out in the correct way (because we are subject to all sorts of conscious and subconscious influences on our thinking which can distort it).

54 My own answers would include:
- that I do not know but which is true: almost everything
- that I know but which is not true: that I can draw a straight line (space is warped)
- that I believe but I do not know: that there may be a personal nature to the nothingness (I can't find him/her)
- that I know but that I do not believe: that I have no concrete existence (I think therefore I am; but who is it who thinks?)
- that I believe but that is not true: that time is constant (it varies with changes through space)
- that is true, but that I do not believe: that there is nothing (I 'know' this to be 'true' on an intellectual and experiential level; but somehow I can't quite bring myself to believe it).

55 A posteriori – based upon observation.

56 A priori – based upon logic building from foundational axioms.

57 David Hume (Hume 1739) was the first philosopher to point out that knowledge statements can be of two different types: 'it is' and 'it ought to be'. 'It ought to be' statements are 'prescriptive' or 'normative' statements made about what we 'ought'

to do. Hume noted that people often try to say what 'ought' to be based upon assertions of what 'is'. However, there is no logical link between the two.

He also differentiated between 'it is' statements based upon deductive knowledge (which can be safely arrived at through deduction), and inductive knowledge (which observes and makes judgements based upon observation). He made the point that inductive knowledge is based upon the belief that nature always behaves in the same way (so, for example, because water flows downhill today, we believe that it has always flowed downhill in the past and always will in the future). Of course we can never be certain that is and will be the case. So inductive and deductive statements are of wholly different types.

Hume's work had a large influence on the subject split of knowledge endeavours into mathematics (it is), sciences (it appears to be) and ethics (it ought to be) during the Enlightenment era.

58　For example, in the West, prior to the Enlightenment, metaphysical knowledge predominated and power was held by the church. After the Enlightenment, inductive, empirical knowledge predominated, and power was held by more technologically industrialised nations. After the two world wars, and in particular the Holocaust, recognition of the destructive potential of 'decontextualised' technology and science generated a reaction and development of the importance of contextualising and subjectivising all knowledge to save it from being appropriated and abused by those in positions of power.

59　In the West in the 20th century, medicine has operated very much as an empirical, scientific, hypothetico-deductive approach which is extremely effective at diagnosing problems from the perspective of 'other' but of less use from the perspective of 'me' or 'we'. Complementary therapies that started to be practised in the West towards the end of the last century tend to do the opposite. It would be good to try to practise in a way that covers both approaches, using each in the appropriate and apposite way.

60　If you are not sure, try to complete the following table for each of the conditions:

Question	Your answer
Are there observable facts about this condition?	
Does the condition require some interpretation of what is 'normal' and 'abnormal'?	
Does the state of mind of the patient or relevant other affect the patient's experience of the condition?	
Does the patient's culture affect his/her understanding and experience of his/her condition?	
Does the patient think that some sort of external forces (like environment, social, spiritual, economic forces) may have been at play in the development of (or his experience of) the condition?	

Question	Your answer
Is the condition in any way 'disabling' for the patient?	

61 For example, we could take a number of different perspectives.

- We could see him as an 'I', and ask him how it feels to smoke, what the meaning and purpose of it is for him, and how it affects his sense of well-being and health. This might open up psychological, cognitive and spiritual approaches to healthcare.
- We could see him as a 'we' and look at the familial and cultural context of his smoking. What pressures is he under, what are the norms for him, what are the narratives and contexts? This might open up narrative, dramatic, familial and cultural approaches to healthcare.
- We could see him as an individual 'other'; examining empirically the effect of smoking on his heart, lungs and blood vessels. We could calculate his risk score of dying from his smoking. This might open up physical, physiological, pharmacological and surgical approaches to care.
- We could see him as part of a wider society of 'others', which we could also examine empirically, looking at historical, sociological, environmental, and behavioural factors at play in his decision to smoke. This might open up societal, environmental, ecological, economic and political approaches to care.

62 By Luke Fildes (public domain art).

63 Some questions might be:

- What does she mean by 'feeling' and how is it 'terrible'?
- Who are the 'all'?
- Why use the imagery of slavery?
- What does 'down' mean, and why is health anything to do with height or depth?
- What is the 'it'? Does she think the cancer has a consciousness or is in some way an agent working against her?
- Why use martial imagery of invasion and destruction?
- How has drink aided or hindered her sense of health?
- Which God, and how might he/she be involved in her health?
- Is the drink an agent, in some way both within and working against her family?
- Why use the imagery of being hooked? Who is the fisherman, and what was the bait?
- What would 'the point' look like for her?

64 With thanks to 'The History of Frenchay Hospital' by James Briggs. Image in the public domain.

65 Image provided under licence by www.photos.com

66 They describe their '4 Cs' theory in which we can generate increasing levels of expertise and complexity with our creativity: creativity as 'mini-c', including personal experiences and insights; 'little-c' including the way we creatively problem solve and express these creations day to day; 'pro-C' including creativity demonstrated by experts in their field; and 'big-C' including major, transformative steps of human creativity which offer everyone a new perspective on existence.

67 Image provided under licence from www.photos.com

68 The theory of cognitive dissonance suggests that it is very uncomfortable for us to hold contradictory ideas or thought patterns. When we feel this discomfort, we feel motivated to do something to stop it. Two opinions, or beliefs, or items of knowledge, are dissonant with each other if they do not fit together; that is, if they are inconsistent, or if, considering only the particular two items, one does not follow from the other (Festinger 1957). We cannot prove or disprove the existence of dissonance, or its effect on creativity. As dissonance is an experiential form of knowledge, by definition it becomes impossible to prove empirically. However, we can look for associative evidence, and there is some evidence to suggest dissonance increases arousal and activity in certain parts of the brain (Festinger 195; Sharot 2009; Van Veen 2009).

69 Festinger 1957; Sharot 2009; Van Veen 2009.

70 Adapted from Wallas 1926.

71 The elements required for convergence seem to be quite different to those required for divergence. Divergence seems to require us to generate and experience a sense of relaxation and distance, so that our subconscious can flow effortlessly. Convergence is a single-minded, effortful process requiring tenacity, objective and analytical testing, and persistent creative effort to put our idea into reality.

So, again, creativity appears to arise from dynamic tension and the relational interplay between different types of knowledge and different types of thinking. As we become explicitly aware of implicit dissonance we start to diverge from that point, looking for possible new ideas, thoughts or actions that might help us regain consonance. When such ideas occur, we converge on them, checking them for usefulness and effectiveness, and planning how to enact them.

This is not so foreign to us as health practitioners. The recent emphasis on empiricism, evidence-based practice, targets and guidelines emphasises the importance of careful analysis, clarity of thought and measurable, effective outcomes in health practice. There is nothing 'wrong' with any of these. We all hope to achieve all of them. However, as practitioners, we are also aware of the importance of being able to imagine what it is like to be the patient, to see the world from his or her perspective, to explore new ways of seeing and managing the problems, and create plans and treatments which will be most effective.

72 When we are confronted by a challenging or new situation, this theory suggests that our brains seem to comb through and pull apart existing memories, sending them to the cortex to be blended with new senses and ideas, before being recomposed and fine-tuned in the cerebellum into prototypes or models for action. What is interesting is that these cerebellar-cortical loops seem to train themselves with practice, becoming more and more efficient at the prototyping process.

73 When confronted with dissonance, the mind seems to comb back subconsciously through previous memories looking for similar patterns and ideas, creating models or prototypes, and testing these models or prototypes against memory to consider how effective they are likely to be. Different researchers have demonstrated different patterns of neural activation, involving different parts of the brain. In truth neuroscience is a long way from definitive answers to how the brain creates. However,

the cerebral cortex may have a role both in storing memories and in generating new ideas, whereas the cerebellum may have a role in coordinating, balancing and fine-tuning prototypes: integrating different inputs from different patterns of activity, from memory and from the senses (Vandervert, Schimpf & Liu 2007). This is similar to the cerebellum's function in controlling, balancing and fine-tuning movement and thought.

74 With thanks to Fabian for his permission. Fabian's work can be seen at http://fabianperez.com

75 Kahneman (2012) suggests we will intuit answers to problems even when we are completely new to the problem. As novices, our intuition is much more likely to be wrong (even though we intuitively feel it is right). This is maybe why we are nervous of using intuition in practice. However, he also demonstrates that intuition becomes safer and more effective as we become more experienced and familiar with the situation.

This is much more like the situation that prevails in our own health practice – in which by definition we are more expert and familiar than others. It seems we may be avoiding using a tool which is fast, effective and not tiring to use.

Kahneman argues that our intuitive thinking can be biased by a number of factors. If we can be aware of these factors, we can be more expert in using our intuition safely and effectively. These factors include the following.

- Always looking for a cause: our intuition wants to make connections, so will look for causes even where the event was a chance event.
- Mistaking plausibility for probability: something may happen. That makes it plausible. But it may be unlikely to happen. That makes it improbable.
- Availability bias: the more emotion generated (e.g. anxiety) when we think about something, the more likely we think it is to occur, probably because our subconscious is making the possibility very 'available' to our intuition.
- Risk aversion: people prefer to avoid loss than to acquire gains.
- Incorrect stereotype: for example, that certain groups are more likely to be more or less prone to certain problems, when in fact there is no difference.
- Framing: the way a question is framed. For example, people are more likely to go for a treatment that has a 90% chance of succeeding than they will for one that has a 10% chance of failing.

76 These principles of expertise are known as (Simon 1973):

- The meaningful encoding principle: experts code and memorise information about the area of expertise more effectively, thereby enabling far more possible avenues and prompts for retrieval of memory.
- The retrieval structure principle: experts develop structures that enable them to retrieve relevant information far more efficiently from long-term memory.
- The speed-up principle: memory encoding and retrieval speeds up and becomes more accurate with practice.

It is not entirely clear why this is, but may be to do with the way we categorise and then represent problems to ourselves. When we are novices, perhaps because we don't fully understand, we use superficial categories built upon immediately apparent but surface features of the information we are studying. However, when we become more expert we recognise and classify information based upon the deep, relational structures of the information. So when we retrieve and represent this information to ourselves, it comes readily attached to a much broader and more relevant range of associated and useful information; which we can apply much more efficiently and effectively.

77 Image provided under licence by www.photos.com

78 Several researchers have shown the importance of a positive sense of mind and well-being for creativity. Isen, Daubman and Nowicki (1987) suggest this is because feeling good makes additional cognitive material available for processing, reduces the focus on our immediate needs or concerns, thereby enabling us to focus more broadly to find a wider scope of elements that might help us address the challenge, and increases our cognitive flexibility, so increasing the probability that diverse cognitive elements will in fact become associated. Fredrickson (2001) suggests that joy and love broaden our repertoire of cognitions and actions, thus enhancing creativity. Various studies have shown divergent thinking is assisted by the development of relaxation (alpha waves) in the brain, the increased activity of the frontal lobe (thought to be important in idea generation) and the temporal lobe (thought to be important for editing and moulding new ideas), sufficient sleep and rest, a positive mood, the presence of joy and love, and the existence of a positive, supportive, encouraging environment.

On the other hand, contrary studies show that, while happiness and a sense of well-being may be important for generating new ideas; negative states of mind like rumination, obsession and even depression (which encourage isolation, rumination and perseveration) can also be useful in creativity.

Lehrer (2012) speculates that while happiness and well-being are useful for generating ideas, they are less useful for putting them into practice. Expert creations take a great deal of effort and perseverance to put them into practice. Things like perseveration, rumination and single-mindedness tend to be characteristics of lower states of mind. This correlates with findings that while drugs that make us relaxed and feel good (such as cannabis) are good for helping us generate new ideas and perspectives; drugs that make us focus or concentrate (such as amphetamines and caffeine) tend to make us more effective and efficient in practical applications. Perhaps they need both the 'ups' and the 'downs' to be really creative, which may account for the higher incidence of bipolar disorder in 'creative' people.

79 Lehrer (2012) cites a number of experiments showing how our creativity and our ability to do hard mental reasoning can be affected by the environment. For example, our ability to look for, and find, creative new ideas and connections is assisted by helping our brains find cognitive ease: such as when taking a hot shower, going for a walk, having a drink or two, being around the colour blue. On the other hand, our ability to test the correctness of our ideas, and make them work in practice, is assisted by putting our brains under slight cognitive strain so that they can focus and stick at the task. For example, students asked to perform reasoning and short-term memory tests in red environments do better than in blue environments, whereas they do worse on imaginative or creative tasks. He also cites interesting examples of how different thinkers and creators use relaxants (such as alcohol or

cannabis) to assist the generation of creative ideas, but use stimulants (such as caffeine or amphetamines) to give them the cognitive strength and resilience to make their creative ideas into reality. It is a delicate balancing act, though: too much relaxation simply leads to unproductive daydreaming, while too much stimulation leads to exhaustion and loss of perspective.

80 In summary:

- Keeping perspective: patients come to us because of dissonance. They are not as healthy as they wish to be. To help our patients we therefore need to co-create better health with them. So we can encourage ourselves and others that creativity is not just possible but essential for effective health practice.

- Dedicating and committing: we will create more effectively if we can become clear about our purpose and dedicated in our intention 'to create better health', not just one a year or one a month, but in every moment, with every patient.

- Practising righteously: if we can set ourselves and our practice up in such a way that we can try different ways of doing things and have opportunities for learning and discovery as we practise, we will have a greater chance of being creative. Guidelines, information and targets can be helpful in focusing our skills down the most effective channels. But we need to balance these by creating space and time for ourselves to think and act differently, trying new things in new ways.

- Becoming mindfully aware: so that we can become immediately aware if we are straying into too much cognitive ease and complacency; or if we are straying into too much cognitive angst, distraction and paralysis. When we are aware we will spot dissonance arising within us, and rush to welcome it as a useful tool (rather than rush to avoid or ignore it as an unwelcome distraction).

- Communicating effectively with ourselves and others: to create we need to create the space, time and environment to allow the creative tensions to emerge and the creative dance to play out. We need to give ourselves and our colleagues the time, space and environment to converge and diverge, and for our convergence and divergence to interplay with each other, creating, modelling and testing new ideas. By consciously creating mental space and time, we give ourselves the confidence and a willingness to take risks and try new things where things are not working, rather than allowing ourselves to be paralysed by distraction or ruminations about all the things that could go wrong.

- Acting skilfully: recognising where we are strong, and where we can become more expert in our creativity. Keeping our minds and bodies as healthy, balanced and poised as possible, so we are ready to embrace dissonance and find integration and balance. Learning continuously, because the more knowledge we have, the more resources our creative mind has to develop new ideas, and the more tools it has to test new ideas against. Practising continuously, so that we can observe ever more complex patterns and associations, because the more complex patterns and associations we are aware of, the more powerful is our springboard for ongoing creativity.

- Dancing expertly: pulling in all the diverse people, technologies, perspectives, states of mind, drives, motivations, hopes, memories, knowledge, thoughts, ideas and actions, looking always to bring them to the point of integrated, harmonic balance: standing out against the nothingness, but in continuous harmony with it.

81 Kolb (1984) suggested we have different learning styles based around a learning cycle. The cycle of learning is:
- concrete experience (CE)
- reflective observation (RO)
- abstract conceptualisation (AC)
- active experimentation (AE)
- back to CE again.

These can be grouped into perceiving activities (experience and conceptualisation) and processing activities (observation and experimentation). Each of us tends to prefer a particular stage on the cycle, and therefore these govern our learning styles:
- Diverging 'Reflectors' (CE/RO) – prefer feeling and watching
- Assimilating 'Theorists' (AC/RO) – prefer watching and thinking
- Converging 'Pragmatists' (AC/AE) – prefer thinking and doing
- Accommodating 'Activists' (CE/AE) – prefer doing and feeling.

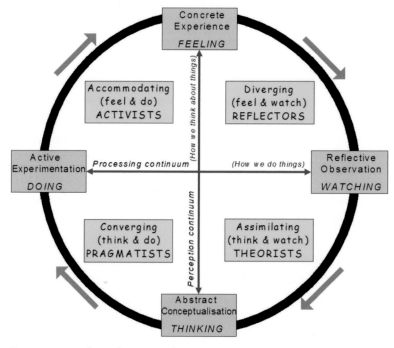

Source: www.brainboxx.co.uk

Gibbs' reflective cycle (Gibbs 1988), commonly used as the basis for clinical supervision, is helpful in that it provides a framework for breaking down different elements of practice and reflecting on them independently, before reintegrating them.
- Stage 1: Description of the event (facts only, no emotions or judgements).
- Stage 2: Feelings (here we can bring out the feelings and emotions that may have arisen).
- Stage 3: Evaluation (a discussion of what went well and less well).
- Stage 4: Analysis (a more detailed discussion of why things went well or badly, and what the various factors at play were).

- Stage 5: Conclusion (a decision about what went well and what would be done differently if it happened again).
- Stage 6: Action (exactly who will do what, where, when and how if the same situation arises in the future).

Rolfe's (Rolfe, Freshwater & Jasper 2001) is similar but more simplified. It just has three stages:

- What: what happened, the effects, consequences, actions, responses, feelings etc.
- So what: what does it mean, what has been learnt (individually and as a group/organisation), implications of relationships, attitudes, cultures and so on.
- Now what: specific actions that need to be done to improve future actions and outcomes.

There are numerous very helpful tools and templates for learning, training and appraisal which are applicable for practitioners everywhere. The Bradford Training Scheme website has a 'Trainers Toolkit' which is a veritable mine of useful stuff. Please look at www.bradfordvts.co.uk

82 According to Eraut (2000) practitioners tend to use a number of different processes in our work:

- assessing patients and situations
- deciding what action to take
- taking a course of action (and modifying this course as needed)
- meta-cognitive watching and monitoring of ourselves, others and the situation developing around us as we work.

As practitioners we also use three different modes of cognition, which we pick and choose depending on the urgency, speed and conditions required:

- Instant/Reflex: this is almost subconscious and automated
- Rapid/Intuitive: which is conscious but only just, as we leap straight from observation to understanding and action without knowing how exactly we got there
- Deliberative/Analytic: which is when we take in the whole picture and put the pieces together before arriving at a decision and action plan.

These processes and cognitive modes interact as in the table below.

Type of Process	Mode of Cognition		
	Instant/Reflex	Rapid/Intuitive	Deliberative/Analytic
Assessment of the situation	Pattern recognition	Rapid interpretation	Prolonged diagnosis Review with discussion and/or analysis
Decision making	Instant response	Intuitive	Deliberative with some analysis or discussion
Overt actions or action scripts	Routinised action	Routines punctuated by rapid decisions	Planned actions with periodic progress reviews
Meta-cognition	Situational awareness	Implicit monitoring Short, reactive reflections	Conscious monitoring of thought and activity Reflection for learning

As we acquire more experience and practice, tasks that required deliberative approaches gradually become more 'routinised' and so we become less aware of them. Thus this knowledge becomes 'tacit' rather than 'explicit'. Tacit knowledge is highly efficient as it gets us where we need to go quickly and effectively.

Tacit knowledge is not without problems. Because we are unaware of it operating, we may not recognise when situations and issues move on, so our short cuts become less and less relevant and secure. Therefore, in professional practice, tacit knowledge tends to be safety-netted by generating and testing hypotheses (e.g. diagnoses) or plans (e.g. management plans) against evidence (e.g. from clinical tests or published evidence) or the views of other people (e.g. colleagues or specialists).

The thing which distinguishes the 'expert' is not just what they know, but also how they use and apply what they know (because their knowledge has been continuously moulded and melded as a result of considerable experience).

The acquisition of tacit knowledge develops best in social contexts, where professionals can discuss and test knowledge with each other. It also requires an open and permissive culture of learning, wherein people feel able to share mistakes as well as successes.

Of particular relevance to health practice, time and thinking interact either in a constructive or destructive way. A certain degree of time shortage forces people to focus more attentively, process more quickly and adopt more intuitive practices. Similarly, a more intuitive approach frees us up to do things faster. More significant time limitations put limitations on meta-cognition, but a slightly less time-pressured environment enables us to meta-process, thus taking into account such factors as self-awareness, awareness of the context and connectedness of problems, awareness of the various ways we can think about the problems, and selection of the most appropriate tools.

Very severe time limitations prevent us even using intuitive actions, as we are forced into almost entirely automated actions, with no time for meta-processing at all. Without some meta-processing, we rapidly lose confidence in our abilities, because we have no feedback against which we can check our actions and decisions. In this situation, the effectiveness and efficiency of our work drops off rapidly.

83 This may appear at first sight to be nonsensical, but if we think about it we know that we can be expert in many things that we do not understand the origins and causes of: for example, speaking our mother tongue, carrying out finely tuned and coordinated movement, complex thinking, and just being conscious.

84 'The Concept of Flow', in Snyder and Lopez (2009).

Bibliography

Abbasi K. Doctors: automatons, technicians, or knowledge brokers? *JRSM*. 2007; **100**(1): 1. Print.

Aked J, Marks N, Cordon C, Thompson S. Five ways to well-being. *Foresight Project on Mental Capital and Wellbeing*. New Economics Foundation; 2008. Web. Available at: www.neweconomics.org/publications/five-ways-well-being-evidence

Alladin A, Alibhai A. Cognitive hypnotherapy for depression: an empirical investigation. *IJCEH*. 2007; **55**(2): 147–66. Print.

Allen RP. *Scripts and Strategies in Hypnotherapy: the complete works.* Carmarthen: Crown House Publishing; 2004. Print.

Ambady N. Surgeons' tone of voice: a clue to malpractice history. *Surgery.* 2002; **132**(1): 5–9. Print.

Amery J. *Children's Palliative Care in Africa.* Oxford: Oxford University Press; 2009. Print.

Anielski M. *The Economics of Happiness: building genuine wealth*. Gabriola, BC: New Society; 2007. Print.

Armstrong D. Space and time in British general practice. *Soc Sci Med.* 1985; **20**(7): 659–66. Print.

Arnetz BB, Horte LG. Suicide patterns among physicians related to other academics as well as to the general populations: results from a national long-term prospective study and a retrospective study. *Acta Psychiatr Scand.* 1987; **75**(2): 139–43. Print.

Balint M. *The Doctor, His Patient, and the Illness.* New York: International Universities; 1957. Print.

Bandura A. Self-efficacy: toward a unifying theory of behavioral change. *Psychol Rev.* 1977; **84**(2): 191–215. Print.

Barsky AJ. Hidden reasons some patients visit doctors. *Ann Intern Med.* 1981; **94**: 492–8. Print.

Beating the Blues®. Web. Available at: www.beatingtheblues.co.uk (accessed 28 October 2011).

Beck DE, Cowan CC. *Spiral Dynamics*. Oxford: Blackwell; 2006. Print.

Beckman HB, Frankel RM. The effect of physician behavior on the collection of data. *Ann Intern Med.* 1984; **101**: 692–6. Print.

Beevers CG, Miller IW. Perfectionism, cognitive bias, and hopelessness as prospective predictors of suicidal ideation. *Suicide and Life-Threatening Behavior.* 2004; **34**(2): 126–37. Print.

Bench M. Open Door Coaching. Web. Available at: www.opendoorcoaching.com. (accessed 17 October 2011). Copyright © 2003 Marcia Bench and Career Coach Institute; reprinted with permission.

Berne E. *Games People Play: the psychology of human relationships*. New York: Grove; 1964. Print.

Betancourt JR, Ananeh-Firempong O. Not me! Doctors, decisions, and disparities in health care: how do we really make decisions? *Cardiovasc Rev Rep*. 2004; **25**(3): n.p. Print.

Better Health. Web. Available at: http://getbetterhealth.com (accessed 17 October 2011).

Black Dog Institute. *Depression*. Black Dog Institute. Web. Available at: www.black doginstitute.org.au (accessed 23 November 2011).

Blanck PD, Buck R, Rosenthal R. *Nonverbal Communication in the Clinical Context*. University Park: Pennsylvania State University Press; 1986. Print.

Blenkiron P. *Stories and Analogies in Cognitive Behavioural Therapy*. Oxford: Wiley Blackwell; 2010. Print.

Block N. How many concepts of consciousness? *Behavioral and Brain Sciences*. 1995; **18**(2):272–8. Print.

BMJ. How much do we know? Clinical Evidence. BMJ. Web. Available at: http://clinical evidence.bmj.com/ceweb/about/knowledge.jsp (accessed 17 October 2011)

Bohm D. *Wholeness and the Implicate Order*. London: Routledge & Kegan Paul; 1981. Print.

Bradford VTS. Trainers' Toolkit. Home. Web. Available at: www.bradfordvts.co.uk (accessed 12 November 2011).

Brantley J. *Calming Your Anxious Mind: how mindfulness and compassion can free you from anxiety, fear, and panic*. Oakland, CA: New Harbinger Publications; 2007. Print.

British Association for Behavioural & Cognitive Psychotherapies. Home Page. Web. Available at: www.babcp.com (accessed 28 October 2011).

British Medical Association. *Doctors' Health*. 8 May 2007. Web. Available at: www.bma. org.uk/doctors_health/doctorshealth.jsp?page=2 (accessed 28 October 2011).

British Medical Association. *Quality and Outcomes Framework, February 2010*. Web. Available at: www.bma.org.uk/employmentandcontracts/independent_contractors/ quality_outcomes_framework/qualityframework10.jsp (accessed 28 October 2011).

Brown D. Evidence-based hypnotherapy for asthma: a critical review. *IJCEH*. 2007; **55**(2): 220–49. Print.

Bruton HJ. Book review: nations and households in economic growth: essays in honor of Moses Abramovitz (Paul A. David, Melvin W. Reder). *Economic Development and Cultural Change*. 1979; **27**(4): 801. Print.

Bstan-'dzin-rgya-mtsho, Hopkins J. *Becoming Enlightened*. New York: Atria; 2009. Print.

Buber M. *I and Thou*. New York: Continuum; 2004. Print.

Buchbinder SB, Wilson M, Melick CF. Estimates of costs of primary care physician turnover. *Am J Managed Care*. 1999; **5**(11): 1431. Print.

Businessballs. *Job Satisfaction Inventory*. Businessballs Free Online Learning for Careers, Work, Management, Business Training and Education. Web. Available at: http:// businessballs.com (accessed 27 October 2011).

Businessballs. Web. Available at: http://businessballs.com (accessed 24 October 2011).

Byrne PS, Long BEL. *Doctors Talking to Patients*. London: HMSO; 1978. Print.

Campbell DT. Blind variation and selective retention in creative thought as in other knowledge processes. *Psychol Rev.* 1960; **67**: 380–400. Print.

Campling P, Haigh R. *Therapeutic Communities: past, present, and future.* London: Jessica Kingsley; 1999. Print.

Campo R. What the body told. *The World in Us: lesbian and gay poetry of the next wave.* New York: Griffin; 2001. N.p. Print.

Caplan F, Caplan T. *The Power of Play.* New York: Doubleday; 1973. Print.

Carroll L, Green RL. *Alice's Adventures in Wonderland; and, through the looking-glass and what Alice found there.* London: Oxford University Press; 1971. Print.

Casey PR, Tyrer P. Personality disorder and psychiatric illness in general practice. *Br J Psychiatry.* 1990; **156**(2): 261–5. Print.

Chomsky N. A minimalist program for linguistic theory. *The View from the Building: essays in honor of Sylvain Bromberger.* Cambridge: MIT; 1993. N.p. Print.

Cole SA, Bird J. *The Medical Interview: the three-function approach.* St. Louis: Mosby; 2000. Print.

Committee on the Use of Complementary and Alternative Medicine by the American Public. *Complementary and Alternative Medicine in the United States.* Washington, DC: National Academies; 2005. Print.

Covey, S. *The 7 Habits Of Highly Effective People.* Free Press; Revised edition 2004.

Cozens J. Doctors, their wellbeing and stress. *BMJ.* 2003; **326**: 670–1. Print.

Csikszentmihalyi M. *Finding Flow: the psychology of engagement with everyday life.* New York: Basic; 1997. Print.

Dalai Lama. *Becoming Enlightened.* London: Rider; 2010. Print.

Dalai Lama, Cutler HC. *The Art of Happiness: a handbook for living.* Audiobook CD. New York: Simon & Schuster Audio; 1998.

Dalai Lama, Hopkins J. *Becoming Enlightened.* New York: Atria; 2009. Print.

Damgaard-Mørch NL, Nielsen LJ, Uldwall SW. [Knowledge and perceptions of complementary and alternative medicine among medical students in Copenhagen]. [Article in Danish] Ugeskr Laeger. 2008; **170**(48): 3941–5. Available in translation at: www.vifab.dk/uk/statistics/medical+students+and+alternative+medicine?

Davison S. Principles of managing patients with personality disorder. *Adv Psychiatr Treat.* 2002; **8**: 1–9. Print.

Deber RB. What role do patients wish to play in treatment decision making? *Arch Intern Med.* 1996; **156**: 1414–20. Print.

de Girolamo G, Reich JH. *Epidemiology of Mental Disorders and Psychosocial Problems: personality disorders.* Geneva: World Health Organization; 1993. Print.

DeLongis A, Folkman S, Lazarus RS. The impact of daily stress on health and mood: psychological and social resources as mediators. *J Pers Soc Psychol.* 1988; **54**(3): 486–95. Print.

Dennett DC. *Consciousness Explained.* London: Penguin; 1993. Print.

Deveugele M, Derese A, van den Brink-Muinen A, *et al.* Consultation length in general practice: cross sectional study in six European countries. *BMJ.* 2002; **325**(7362): 472. Print.

Dewey J. *How We Think.* Boston: D.C. Heath & Co; 1910. Print.

Dickinson E, Franklin RW. *The Poems of Emily Dickinson*. Cambridge, MA: Belknap of Harvard University Press; 1998. Print.

Digman JM. Personality structure: emergence of the five-factor model. *Annu Rev Psychology*. 1990; **41**(1): 417–40. Print.

DiMatteo M, Robin CD, Sherbourne RD, *et al*. Physicians' characteristics influence patients' adherence to medical treatment: results from the Medical Outcomes Study. *Health Psychol*. 1993; **12**(2): 93–102. Print.

DOH. *Improving Access to Psychological Therapies (IAPT) Programme: computerised Cognitive Behavioural Therapy (cCBT) implementation guidance*. Department of Health, UK; March 2007. Web. Available at: www.dh.gov.uk/en/Publicationsand statistics/Publications/PublicationsPolicyAndGuidance/DH_073470

DOH. *Delivering Care, Improving Outcomes for Patients*. Quality and Outcomes Framework; 8 February 2010.

DOH. *Mental Health and Ill Health in Doctors*. London: Crown Publishing; 2008. Department of Health. Web. Available at: www.dh.gov.uk/en/Publicationsandstatistics/ Publications/PublicationsPolicyAndGuidance/DH_083066.

DOH. *Mental Health Policy Implementation Guide: adult acute inpatient care provision*. Department of Health (UK); 2002. Web. Available at: www.positive-options.com/ news/downloads/DoH_-_Adult_Acute_In-patient_Care_Provision_-_2002.pdf.

DOH. *The GP Patient Survey: general information*. The GP Patient Survey. UK Department of Health; 2010. Web. Available at: www.gp-patient.co.uk/info

Doran T. Effect of financial incentives on incentivised and non-incentivised clinical activities: longitudinal analysis of data from the UK Quality and Outcomes Framework. *BMJ*. 2011; **342**: 590–8. Print.

Dowson JH, Grounds A. *Personality Disorders: recognition and clinical management*. Cambridge: Cambridge University Press; 1995. Print.

Dunnette MD, Hough LM, Triandis HC. *Handbook of Industrial and Organizational Psychology*. Palo Alto, CA: Consulting Psychologists; 1990. Print.

Durkheim É, Cladis CS. *The Elementary Forms of Religious Life*. Oxford: Oxford University Press; 2001. Print.

Durojave OC. Health screening: is it always worth doing? *The Internet Journal of Epidemiology*. 2009; **7**(1): n.p. Print.

Easterlin RA. Does economic growth improve the human lot? Some empirical evidence. In: David PA, Reder MW, editors. *Nations and Households in Economic Growth: essays in honor of Moses Abramovitz*. New York: Academic Press; 1974. Print.

Edelman GM, Mountcastle VB. *The Mindful Brain: cortical organization and the group-selective theory of higher brain function*. Cambridge: MIT; 1978. Print.

Edelman GM, Tononi G. *A Universe of Consciousness: how matter becomes imagination*. New York, NY: Basic; 2000. Print.

Ely JW, Osheroff JA, Ebell M. Analysis of questions asked by family doctors regarding patient care. *BMJ*. 1997; **319**: 358–61. Print.

Epstein RM. Mindful practice. *JAMA*. 1999; **292**(9): 833. Print.

Eraut M. Non-formal learning and tacit knowledge in professional work. *Br J Educ Psychol*. 2000; **70**(1): 113–36. Print.

Erickson HC, Tomlin EM, Price Swain MA. *Modeling and Role Modeling: a theory and paradigm for nursing.* Englewood Cliffs, NJ: Prentice-Hall; 1983. Print.

Ericsson KA. *The Cambridge Handbook of Expertise and Expert Performance.* Cambridge: Cambridge University Press; 2006. Print.

Ernst E. Obstacles to research in complementary and alternative medicine. *Med J Aust.* 2003; **179**(6): 279–80. Print.

Evans R. Releasing time to care: Productive Ward, survey results. *Nurs Times.* 2007; **10**(Suppl. 16): S6–9.

Eve R. *PUNs and DENs: discovering learning needs in general practice.* Oxford: Radcliffe Medical Press; 2003. Print.

Everett DL. *Don't Sleep, There Are Snakes: life and language in the Amazonian jungle.* New York: Pantheon; 2008. Print.

FearFighter. Panic & Phobia Treatment. CCBT Limited Healthcare online. Web. Available at: www.fearfighter.com

Festinger L. *A Theory of Cognitive Dissonance.* California: Stanford University Press; 1957. Print.

Figusch Z, editor. *From One-to-one Psychodrama to Large Group Socio-psychodrama: more writings from the arena of Brazilian psychodrama.* Figusch; 2009. Print.

Finke RA, Ward TB, Smith SM. *Creative Cognition: theory, research, and applications.* Cambridge, MA: MIT; 1996. Print.

Firth-Cozens J. Doctors, their wellbeing, and their stress. *BMJ.* 2003; **326**: 670–1. Print.

Flett G. York researcher finds that perfectionism can lead to imperfect health. *York's Daily Bulletin.* Toronto, Canada: York University; June 2004. Print.

Flood GD. *An Introduction to Hinduism.* New York, NY: Cambridge University Press; 1996. Print.

Flynn JR. *What Is Intelligence: beyond the Flynn Effect.* Expanded paperback ed. Cambridge: Cambridge University Press; 2009. Web. http://en.wikipedia.org/wiki/International_Standard_Book_Number

Foresight Project. *Mental Capital and Wellbeing: making the most of ourselves in the 21st century.* The Foresight Project. The Government Office for Science: London; 2008. Web.

Foucault M. *History of Madness.* London: Routledge; 2006. Print.

Fowler KA, Lilienfield SO, Patrick CJ. Detecting psychopathy from thin slices of behaviour. *Psychol Assess.* 2009; **21**: 68–78. Print.

Frackowiak RSJ, Ashburner JT, Penny WD *et al. Human Brain Function.* 2nd ed. San Diego, California: Academic Press; 2004. Print.

Frankel RM. From sentence to sequence: understanding the medical encounter through microinteractional analysis. *Discourse Processes.* 1984; **7**(2): 135–70. Print.

Fredrickson BL. The role of positive emotions in positive psychology: the broaden-and-build theory of positive emotions. *Am Psychol.* 2001; **56**(3): 218–26. Print.

Gabora L. The origin and evolution of culture and creativity. *Journal of Memetics.* 1997; **1**(1): n.p. Print.

Gardner, H. *Frames of Mind: The Theory of Multiple Intelligences.* 3rd ed. Basic Books, 2011. Print.

Gettier EL. Is justified true belief knowledge. *Analysis.* 1963. **23**: 121–3. Print.

Gibbs G. *Learning by Doing: a guide to teaching and learning methods.* [London]: FEU; 1988. Print.

Gilbert DT. *Stumbling on Happiness.* New York: Vintage; 2007. Print.

Gilbert E. *Eat, Pray, Love: one woman's search for everything.* New York: Penguin; 2006. Print.

Giles J. *No Self to Be Found: the search for personal identity.* Lanham: University of America; 1997. Print.

Gillon R. Medical ethics: 'four principles plus attention to scope'. *BMJ.* 1994; **309**: 184. Print.

Glaser BG, Strauss AS. *Awareness of Dying.* Chicago: Aldine Pub.; [1965]. Reprint 2005. Print.

GMC. *Disciplinary Decisions.* Rep. General Medical Council. Web. Available at: www.gmc-uk.org/concerns/hearings_and_decisions/fitness_to_practise_decisions.asp

GMC. *Good Medical Practice.* Rep. General Medical Council UK, 2006. Web. Available at: www.gmc-uk.org/guidance/good_medical_practice.asp

GMC. *Printable Documents.* Summer 2009. Web. Available at: www.gmc-uk.org/concerns/printable_documents.asp

Goldberg LR. The structure of phenotypic personality traits. *Am Psychol.* 1993; **48**: 26–34. Print.

GP Online. *A Registrar Survival Guide . . . setting up your consulting room.* GP Online. 2010. Web. Available at: www.gponline.com/Education/article/1037805/a-registrar-survival-guide-setting-consulting-room (accessed 4 November 2010).

GP Training Net. *Consultation Theory.* Web. Available at: http://gptraining.net (accessed 12 November 2011).

Grant J, Crawley J. *Transference and Projection: mirrors to the self.* Buckingham: Open University; 2002. Print.

Greene B. *The Elegant Universe: superstrings, hidden dimensions, and the quest for the ultimate theory.* London: Vintage; 2005. Print.

Greenhalgh T, Hurwitz B, editors. *Narrative Based Medicine: dialogue and discourse in clinical practice.* London: BMJ; 2002. Print.

Grimshaw GM, Stanton T. Tobacco cessation interventions for young people. *Cochrane Database Syst Rev.* 2006; **4**: CD003289. Print.

Haigh R. Modern milieux: therapeutic community solutions to acute ward problems. *The Psychiatrist.* 2002; **26**: 380–2. Print.

Haigh R. The quintessence of a therapeutic environment: five universal qualities. In: Campling P, Haigh R, editors. *Therapeutic Communities: past, present and future.* London: Jessica Kingsley; 1999. pp. 246–57. Print.

Hakeda YS. *Kukai: major works.* New York: Columbia University Press; 1972. Print.

Hall ET. *The Hidden Dimension.* Garden City, NY: Doubleday; 1966. Print.

Hammond DC. Review of the efficacy of clinical hypnosis with headaches and migraines. *IJCEH.* 2007; **55**(2): 207–19. Print.

Handy CB. *Gods of Management: the changing work of organizations.* New York: Oxford University Press; 1995. Print.

Handy CB. *Understanding Organisations.* Harmondsworth, Middlesex: Penguin; [1976] 1985. Print.

Hawking SW. *A Brief History of Time: from the big bang to black holes.* Toronto: Bantam; 1988. Print.

Health Foundation. *Evidence: helping people help themselves. A review of the evidence considering whether it is worthwhile to support self-management.* Health Foundation; May 2011. Web. Available at: www.health.org.uk/publications/evidence-helping-people-help-themselves

Health Talk Online. *Shared Decision Making.* Healthtalkonline. DOH. Web. Available at: www.healthtalkonline.org/Improving_health_care/shared_decision_making (accessed April 2011).

Hecht MA, LaFrance M. How (fast) can I help you? Tone of voice and telephone operator efficiency in interactions. *J Appl Soc Psychol.* 1995; **25**(23): 2086–98. Print.

Hélie S, Sun R. Incubation, insight, and creative problem solving: a unified theory and a connectionist model. *Psychol Rev.* 2010; **117**(3): 994–1024. Print.

Helman CG. Disease versus illness in general practice. *J R Coll Gen Pract.* 1981; **31**: 548–62. Print.

Hendrich A, Chow MP, Skierczynski BA, Lu Z. A 36-hospital time and motion study: how do medical-surgical nurses spend their time? *Perm J.* 2008; **12**(3): 25–34. Print.

Henning K, Ey S, Shaw D. Perfectionism, the impostor phenomenon and psychological adjustment in medical, dental, nursing and pharmacy students. *Med Educ.* 1998; **32**(5): 456–64. Print.

Hermans HJM, Gieser T. *Handbook of Dialogical Self Theory.* Cambridge: Cambridge University Press; 2011. Print.

Hermans HJM, Kempen HJG. *The Dialogical Self: meaning as movement.* San Diego: Academic; 1993. Print.

Heron J. A six-category intervention analysis. *Br J Guidance & Counselling.* 1976; **4**(2): 143–55. Print.

Herzberg F. *The Motivation to Work.* New York: Wiley; 1959. Print.

Hinduism Today. *Join the Hindu Renaissance.* Hinduism Today Magazine. Web. Available at: www.hinduismtoday.com (accessed 14 November 2011).

Hilbert D, Cohn-Vossen S. *Geometry and the Imagination.* 2nd ed. London: Chelsea Publishing Company; 1990. Print.

Hofstadter DR. *Gödel, Escher, Bach.* Harmondsworth: Penguin; 1980. Print.

Hume D. *A Treatise of Human Nature; being an attempt to introduce the experimental method of reasoning into moral subjects.* Cleveland: World Pub.; [1739] 1962. Print.

Hutton W. *The State We're In.* London: Jonathan Cape; 1995. Print.

Hymes J. editor. *The Child under Six.* London: Consortium; 1994. Print.

Ignatow D. *Against the Evidence: selected poems, 1934–1994.* [Middletown, Conn.]: Wesleyan University Press; 1993. Print.

Internet Encyclopedia of Philosophy. *Time.* Internet Encyclopedia of Philosophy. Web. Available at: www.iep.utm.edu/time (accessed 14 November 2011).

Isaksen SG, Treffinger DJ. *Creative Problem Solving: the basic course.* Buffalo, NY: Bearly; 1985. Print.

Isen A, Daubman KA, Nowicki GP. Positive affect facilitates creative problem solving. *J Pers Soc Psychol.* 1987; **52**(6): 1122–31. Print.

Ivancevich JM, Matteson MT. Stress and work: a managerial perspective. In: Quick JC, Bhagat RS, Dalton JE, Quick JD, editors. *Work Stress: health care systems in the workplace*. New York: Praeger; 1980. pp. 27–49. Print.

James W. *The Principles of Psychology*. Charleston, SC: BiblioLife; 2010. Print.

Juran JM, Gryna FM. *Juran's Quality Control Handbook*. New York: McGraw-Hill; 1988. Print.

Kabat-Zinn J. *Full Catastrophe Living: using the wisdom of your body and mind to face stress, pain, and illness*. New York, NY: Dell Pub., a Division of Bantam Doubleday Dell Pub. Group; 1991. Print.

Kahn RL, Byosiere P. Stress in organizations. In: Dunnette MD, Hough LM, editors. *Handbook of Industrial and Organizational Psychology, Vol. 3*. Palo Alto, CA: Consulting Psychologists Press; 1992. pp. 571–650. Print.

Kahneman D. *Thinking, Fast and Slow*. New York: Penguin; 2012. Print.

Kandel ER, Schwartz JM, Jessell TM. *Principles of Neural Science*. New York: McGraw-Hill, Health Professions Division; 2000. Print.

Kant I. *Groundwork for the Metaphysics of Morals*. New Haven: Yale University Press; 2002. Print.

Kaufman JC, Beghetto RA. Beyond big and little: the Four C Model of Creativity. *Rev Gen Psychology*. 2009; **13**: 1–12. Print.

Keating T. Centering Prayer. Web. Available at: www.centeringprayer.com (accessed 12 November 2011).

King LS. *Medical Thinking: a historical preface*. Princeton, NJ: Princeton University Press; 1982. Print.

Kleinke CL, Peterson TR, Rutledge TR. Effects of self-generated facial expressions on mood. *J Pers Soc Psychol*. 1998; **74**(1): 272–9. Print.

Kleinman A. *Patients and Healers in the Context of Culture: an exploration of the borderland between anthropology, medicine, and psychiatry*. Berkeley: University of California; 1980. Print.

Ko U. Ananda. *Beyond Self: 108 Korean Zen poems*. Berkeley, CA: Parallax; 1997. Print.

Koch R. *The Natural Laws of Business: applying the theories of Darwin, Einstein, and Newton to achieve business success*. New York: Currency/Doubleday; 2001. Print.

Koestler A. *The Ghost in the Machine*. London: Hutchinson; 1967. Print.

Kolb DA. *Experiential Learning: experience as the source of learning and development*. Englewood Cliffs, NJ: Prentice-Hall; 1984. Print.

Kornfield J. *Buddha's Little Instruction Book*. London: Rider & Co; 1996. Print.

Kotter JP. *Leading Change*. Boston, MA: Harvard Business School; 1996. Print.

Kumar M. *Quantum: Einstein, Bohr, and the great debate about the nature of reality*. New York: W.W. Norton; 2009. Print.

Kurtz SM, Silverman J, Draper J. *Teaching and Learning Communication Skills in Medicine*. Oxford: Radcliffe Publishing; 2005. Print.

Lalor D. *Creating a Therapeutic Environment. Counselling in Perth, Western Australia*. Cottesloe Counselling Centre. Web. Available at: www.cottesloecounselling.com.au (accessed 24 October 2011).

Lazarus RS, Folkman S. *Stress, Appraisal, and Coping*. New York: Springer; 1984.

Launer J. *Narrative-based Primary Care: a practical guide*. Oxford: Radcliffe Medical Press; 2002. Print.

Légaré F, Ratté S, Stacey D, *et al.* Interventions for improving the adoption of shared decision making by healthcare professionals. *Cochrane Database Syst Rev.* 2011; **10**: CD001431. Web.

Lehrer J. *Imagine: how creativity works*. Edinburgh: Canongate; 2012. Print.

Levensky E, Forcehimes A, Beitz K. Motivational interviewing: an evidence-based approach to counseling helps patients follow treatment recommendations. *Am J Nurs.* 2007; **107**(10): 50–8. Print.

Lewin S, Skea Z, Entwistle V, *et al.* Effects of interventions to promote a patient-centred approach in clinical consultations. *Cochrane Database Syst Rev.* 2001; **4**: CD00326. Web.

Lewin SA, Skea Z, Entwistle VA, *et al.* Interventions for providers to promote a patient-centred approach in clinical consultations. *Cochrane Database Syst Rev.* 2012; **12**: CD003267. Print.

Linehan M. *Cognitive Behavioural Treatment of Borderline Personality Disorder*. London: Guildford; 1993. Print.

Linn LS, Yager J, Cope D, Leake B. Health status, job satisfaction, job stress, and life satisfaction among academic and clinical faculty. *JAMA.* 1985; **254**(19): 2775–82. Print.

Living Life to the Full. *Free Online Skills Course*. Living Life to the Full. Web. Available at: www.llttf.com (accessed 28 October 2011).

Locke J, Bassett T, Holt E. *An Essay Concerning Humane Understanding: in four books*. London: Printed by Eliz. Holt for Thomas Basset; 1690. Print.

Mackenzie RA. *The Time Trap*. New York: AMACOM; 1972. Print.

Maslach C, Schaufeli W, Leiter M. Job burnout. *Annu Rev Psychol.* 2001; **52**: 397–422. Web.

Maslow AH. A theory of human motivation. *Psychol Rev.* 1943; **50**(4): 370–96. Print.

Maslow AH. *The Farther Reaches of Human Nature*. New York: Penguin; 1976. Print.

May R. *The Courage to Create*. London: Collins; 1976. Print.

McCambridge J. Motivational interviewing is equivalent to more intensive treatment, superior to placebo, and will be tested more widely. *Evidence-Based Mental Health.* 2004. **7**(2): 52. Print.

McKinlay JB, Potter DA, Feldman DA. Non-medical influences on medical decision-making. *Soc Sci Med.* 1996; **42**(5): 769–76. Print.

McQuaid JR, Carmona PE. *Peaceful Mind: using mindfulness and cognitive behavioral psychology to overcome depression*. Oakland, CA: New Harbinger; 2004. Print.

McVicar A. Workplace stress in nursing: a literature review. *J Adv Nurs.* 2003; **44**(6): 633–42. Print.

Melville A. Job satisfaction in general practice: implications for prescribing. *Soc Sci Med. Part A: Medical Psychology & Medical Sociology.* 1980; **14**(6): 495–9. Print.

Mitchley SE. The medical interview: the three-function approach. *Postgrad Med J.* 1992; **68**(799): 397–8. Print.

MoodGYM. Welcome. Web. Available at: www.moodgym.anu.edu.au (accessed 28 October 2011).

Moran P. *Antisocial Personality Disorder*. London: Gaskell; 1999. Print.

Morrison T. *Staff Supervision in Social Care: making a real difference for staff and service users*. Brighton: Pavilion; 2005. Print.

National Institute for Health and Care Excellence. *Anxiety: management of anxiety (panic disorder, with or without agoraphobia, and generalised anxiety disorder) in adults in primary, secondary and community care*. NICE. March 2011. Web. Available at: http://guidance.nice.org.uk/CG22

National Institute for Health and Care Excellence. *Brief Interventions and Referral for Smoking Cessation in Primary Care and Other Settings*. NICE. 2006. Web. Available at: www.nice.org.uk/nicemedia/pdf/SMOKING-ALS2_FINAL.pdf

National Institute for Health and Care Excellence. *Cognitive Behavioural Therapy for the Management of Common Mental Health Problems*. NICE. December 2010. Web. Available at: www.nice.org.uk/usingguidance/commissioningguides/cognitivebehavioural therapyservice/cbt.jsp

National Institute for Health and Care Excellence. *Computerised Cognitive Behaviour Therapy for Depression and Anxiety: review of Technology Appraisal 51*. NICE. February 2006. Web. Available at: www.nice.org.uk/nicemedia/pdf/TA097guidance.pdf

Neighbour R. *The Inner Consultation: how to develop an effective and intuitive consulting style*. Lancaster: MTP; 1987. Print.

NHS Centre for Reviews. *Effectiveness Matters: counselling in primary care*. 2001; **5**(2): n.p. Print.

NHS Direct. *Decision Aids*. NHS Direct. Web. Available at: www.nhsdirect.nhs.uk/decisionaids.

NHS Institute for Innovation and Improvement. *Releasing Time to Care: the productive ward*. 2007. Available at: www.institute.nhs.uk/quality_and_value/productivity_series/productive_ward.html.

Noonuccal, Oodgeroo. *My People*. 3rd ed. Milton, QA: The Jacaranda Press; 1990. Print.

Ogedegbe G. Labeling and hypertension: it is time to intervene on its negative consequences. *Hypertension*. 2010; **56**(3): 344–5. Print.

O'Hara LA. Creativity and intelligence. In: Sternberg RJ, editor. *Handbook of Creativity*. Cambridge University Press; 1999. Print.

Open Door Coaching. *Job Satisfaction Inventory*. Open Door Coaching. Web. Available at: www.opendoorcoaching.com/PDF%20files/Job%20Satisfaction%20Inventory. PDF (accessed 24 October 2011).

Orwell G. *Nineteen Eighty-four, a novel*. New York: Harcourt, Brace; 1949. Print.

'Overcoming' series. Constable & Robinson Publishers. Web. Available at: www.over coming.co.uk

Paice E, Moss F. How important are role models in making good doctors. *BMJ*. 2002; **325**: 707. Print.

Patient.co.uk. *Significant Event Analysis*. Health Information and Advice, Medicines Guide, Patient.co.uk. Web. Available at: http://patient.co.uk (accessed 24 October 2011).

Patrick CJ, Craig KD, Prkachin KM. Observer judgments of acute pain: facial action determinants. *J Pers Soc Psych*. 1986; **50**(6): 1291–8. Print.

Pendleton D, Schofield T, Tate P, Havelock P. *The Consultation: an approach to learning and teaching*. Oxford: Oxford University Press; 1984. Print.

Penrose R. *The Emperor's New Mind: concerning computers, minds, and the laws of physics*. Oxford: Oxford University Press; 1989. Print.

Pepler D J. Play and divergent thinking. In: Pepler DJ, Rubin KH. *The Play of Children: current theory and research*. Basel; New York: Karger; 1982. Print.

Pepler DJ, Rubin KH, editors. *The Play of Children: current theory and research*. Basel; New York: Karger; 1982. Print.

Prkachin KM. Dissociating spontaneous and deliberate expressions of pain: signal detection analyses. *Pain*. 1992; **51**(1): 57–65. Print.

Prochaska JO, DiClemente CC. *The Transtheoretical Approach: crossing traditional boundaries of therapy*. Malabar, Florida: R. E. Krieger; 1994. Print.

Proshansky H. The field of environmental psychology. *Handbook of Environmental Psychology*. New York: Wiley; 1987. Print.

Proshansky H, Fabian A, Kaminoff R. Place-identity: physical world socialization of the self. *J Environ Psychol*. 1983; **3**(1): 57–83. Print.

Quakers. *Quaker Faith & Practice: the book of Christian discipline of the yearly meeting of the Religious Society of Friends (Quakers) in Britain*. London: Yearly Meeting of the Religious Society of Friends (Quakers) in Britain; 2009. Print.

Reuler JB, Nardone DA. Role modeling in medical education. *West J Med*. 1994; **160**(4): 335–7. Print.

Rolfe G, Freshwater D, Jasper M. *Critical Reflection for Nursing and the Helping Professions: a user's guide*. Houndmills, Basingstoke, Hampshire: Palgrave; 2001. Print.

Rossman J. *Industrial Creativity; the psychology of the inventor*. New Hyde Park, NY: University; 1964. Print.

Roter DL, Frankel RM, Hall JA, Sluyter D. The expression of emotion through nonverbal behavior in medical visits. Mechanisms and outcomes. *J Gen Intern Med*. 2006; **21**(Suppl. 1): S28–34. Print.

Sackett DL, Rosenberg WM, Gray JA, *et al*. Evidence based medicine: what it is and what it isn't. *BMJ*. 1996; **312**: 71–2. Print.

Sandman, L, Munthe C. Shared decision making, paternalism and patient choice. *Health Care Anal*. 2010; **18**(1): 60–84. Print.

Schegloff EA, Jefferson G, Sacks H. The preference for self-correction in the organization of repair in conversation. *Language*. 1977; **53**: 361–82. Print.

Schön DA. *The Reflective Practitioner: how professionals think in action*. Aldershot: Ashgate; [1983] 2002. Print.

Schwarz, B. *The Paradox of Choice: why more is less*. HarperCollins; New edition; 2005. Print.

Searle JR. *Mind: a brief introduction*. Oxford: Oxford University Press; 2004. Print.

Segal Z, Williams JM, Teasdale J. *Mindfulness-Based Cognitive Therapy for Depression: a new approach to preventing relapse*. New York: Guildford; 2001. Print.

Seligman MEP. *Authentic Happiness: using the new positive psychology to realize your potential for lasting fulfillment*. New York: Free; 2002. Print.

Sharot T, De Martino B, Dolan RJ. Neural activity predicts attitude change in cognitive dissonance. *Nature Neuroscience*. 2009; **29**(12): 3760–5. Print.

Silverman J, Kurtz SM, Draper J. *Skills for Communicating with Patients*. 3rd ed. London: Radcliffe Publishing; 2013. Print.

Simon HA. The mind's eye in chess. In: Chase WG, editor. *Visual Information Processing.* New York: Academic; 1973. Print.

Simon P, Garfunkel A. *The Sounds of Silence.* Columbia, released 1965. CD.

Simonton DK. Creativity, leadership, and chance. In: Sternberg RJ, editor. *The Nature of Creativity.* Cambridge: Cambridge University Press; 1988. Print.

Smith HW. *The 10 Natural Laws of Successful Time and Life Management: proven strategies for increased productivity and inner peace.* New York, NY: Warner; 2003. Print.

Snyder CR, Lopez SJ, editors. *Handbook of Positive Psychology.* Oxford: Oxford University Press; 2009. Print.

Soria R, Legido A, Escolano C. A randomised controlled trial of motivational interviewing for smoking cessation. *Br J Gen Pract.* 2006; **1**(56): 531. Print.

Sowa JF. 'Representing knowledge soup in language and logic'. Available online at: www. jfsowa.com/talks/souprepr.htm

Sternberg RJ. *Beyond IQ: A Triarchic Theory of Intelligence.* Cambridge: Cambridge University Press; 1985.

Stewart I, Joines V. *TA Today: a new introduction to transactional analysis.* Nottingham: Lifespace Pub.; 1987. Print.

Stewart M, Roter D. *Communicating with Medical Patients.* Newbury Park: Sage Publications; 1989. Print.

Stiglitz JE, Sen A, Fitoussi J-P. *Report by the Commission on the Measurement of Economic Performance and Social Progress.* Paris: Commission; 2009. Print.

Stott NC, Davis RH. The exceptional potential in each primary care consultation. *J R Coll Gen Pract.* 1979; **29**: 201–5. Print.

Suzuki DT. *Essays in Zen Buddhism, third series.* London: Published for the Buddhist Society by Rider; 1958. Print.

Suzuki S, Dixon T. *Zen Mind, Beginner's Mind.* New York: Walker/Weatherhill; 1970. Print.

Tarski A. *Logic, Semantics, Metamathematics; papers from 1923 to 1938.* Oxford: Clarendon; 1956. Print.

Taylor D, Bury M. Chronic illness, expert patients and care transition. *Sociology of Health & Illness.* 2007; **29**(1): 27–45. Print.

Tellegen A, Lykken DT, Bouchard TJ, *et al.* Personality similarity in twins reared apart and together. *J Pers Soc Psychol.* 1988; **54**(6): 1031–9. Print.

Thich Nhat Hanh, Mobi Ho, Vo-Dinh Mai. *Miracle of Mindfulness: an introduction.* Boston: Beacon; 1975. Print.

Top Nursing Colleges. *Nursing Theories and Sub-theories.* Top Nursing Colleges. Web. Available at: www.topnursingcolleges.com/nur/nursing-theories-and-sub-theories. html (accessed 12 November 2011).

Tsao L. How much do we know about the importance of play in child development. *Childhood Educ.* Summer 2002. Findarticles.com. Web. Available at: http://findarticles. com/p/articles/mi_qa3614/is_200207/ai_n9147500

Tuckett D, Boulton M, Olson C, Williams A. *Meetings between Experts: an approach to sharing ideas in medical consultations.* London: Tavistock, 1985. Print.

Ubel PA, Angott AM, Zikmund-Fischer BJ. Physicians recommend different treatment for patients than they would choose for themselves. *Arch Intern Med.* 2011; **171**(18): 630–4. Print.

Ulrich RS. How design impacts wellness. *Healthc Forum J.* 1992; **35**(5): 20–5. Print.

Upton J. *Comments.* FearFighter for Panic and Anxiety. Web. Available at: www.fear fighter.com (accessed 28 October 2011).

US National Cancer Institute. *Cancer Screening Overview (PDQ®).* US National Cancer Institute. Web. Available at: www.cancer.gov/cancertopics/pdq/screening/ overview/HealthProfessional/page1 (accessed 24 October 2011).

Van Ham I, Verhoeven A, Groenier K, Groothoff J and De Haan J. Job satisfaction among general practitioners: A systematic literature review. *Eur J Gen Pract.* 2006, **12**(4): 174–80. (doi:10.1080/13814780600994376)

Van Veen V, Krug MK, Scooler JW, Carter CS. Neural activity predicts attitude change in cognitive dissonance. *Nature Neuroscience.* 2009; **12**(11): 1469–74. Print.

Vandervert L, Schimpf P, Liu H. How working memory and the cerebellum collaborate to produce creativity and innovation. *Creativity Res J.* 2007; **19**(1): 1–18. Print.

Various. Evidence based practice in clinical hypnosis. *IJCEH.* 2007; **55**(2): n.p. Print.

Walker L. *Consulting with NLP: Neuro-linguistic Programming in the medical consultation.* Oxford: Radcliffe Medical Press; 2002. Print.

Wallas G. *The Art of Thought.* New York: Harcourt, Brace; 1926. Print.

Warren KS. *Coping with the Biomedical Literature: a primer for the scientist and the clinician.* New York, NY: Praeger; 1981. Print.

Waskett C. An integrated approach to introducing and maintaining supervision: the 4S Model. *Nurs Times.* 2009; **105**(17): 24–6. Print.

Weisberg RW. *Creativity: beyond the myth of genius.* New York: W.H. Freeman; 1993. Print.

West C. Against our will: male interruptions of females in cross-sex conversation. *Annals of the New York Academy of Sciences.* 1979 (Language, Sex); **327**(1): 81–96. Print.

White M. *Maps of Narrative Practice.* New York: W.W. Norton & Co; 2007. Print.

White M, Epston D. *Narrative Means to Therapeutic Ends.* New York: Norton; 1990. Print.

Wilber K. *A Brief History of Everything.* Boston, MA: Shambhala; 2007. Print.

Wilber K. An integral theory of consciousness. *J Consciousness Stud.* 1997; **4**(1): 71–92. Print.

Williams CJ, Garland A. Cognitive-behavioural therapy assessment model for use in clinical practice. *Adv Psych Treat.* 2002; **8**: 172–79. Print.

Williams ES, Konrad TR. Physician, practice, and patient characteristics related to primary care physician physical and mental health: results from the Physician Worklife Study. *Health Services Res.* 2002; **37**(1): 119–41. Print.

Williams ES, Konrad TR, Scheckler WE, *et al.* Understanding physicians' intentions to withdraw from practice: the role of job satisfaction, job stress, mental and physical health. *Health Care Manage Rev.* 2010; **35**(2): 105–15. Web.

Wilson PM, Kendall S, Brooks F. The Expert Patients Programme: a paradox of patient empowerment and medical dominance. *Health & Social Care in the Community.* 2007; **15**(5): 426–38. Web.

Yovel G, Kanwisher N. Face perception: domain specific, not process specific. *Neuron.* 2004; **44**(5): 889–98. Print.

Zhong E, Kenward K, Sheets V, *et al.* Probation and recidivism: remediation among disciplined nurses in six states. *Am J Nurs.* 2009; **109**(3): 48–57. Print.

CPD with Radcliffe

You can now use a selection of our books to achieve CPD (Continuing Professional Development) points through directed reading.

We provide a free online form and downloadable certificate for your appraisal portfolio. Look for the CPD logo and register with us at: www.radcliffehealth.com/cpd

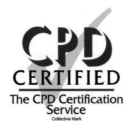